In Clinical Practice

Taking a practical approach to clinical medicine, this series of smaller reference books is designed for the trainee physician, primary care physician, nurse practitioner and other general medical professionals to understand each topic covered. The coverage is comprehensive but concise and is designed to act as a primary reference tool for subjects across the field of medicine.

David T. Huang • Travis Prinzi
Sonja Kreckel
Editors

Cardiac Electrophysiology in Clinical Practice

Second Edition

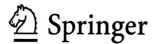

Editors
David T. Huang
Department of Medicine
Cardiology, University of
Rochester Medical Center
Rochester, NY, USA

Travis Prinzi
University of Rochester
Rochester, NY, USA

Sonja Kreckel
Clinical Cardiology
University of Rochester Medical Center
Rochester, NY, USA

ISSN 2199-6652   ISSN 2199-6660 (electronic)
In Clinical Practice
ISBN 978-3-031-41478-7   ISBN 978-3-031-41479-4 (eBook)
https://doi.org/10.1007/978-3-031-41479-4

© The Editor(s) (if applicable) and The Author(s), under exclusive license to Springer Nature Switzerland AG 2023, Springer-Verlag London 2015

This work is subject to copyright. All rights are solely and exclusively licensed by the Publisher, whether the whole or part of the material is concerned, specifically the rights of translation, reprinting, reuse of illustrations, recitation, broadcasting, reproduction on microfilms or in any other physical way, and transmission or information storage and retrieval, electronic adaptation, computer software, or by similar or dissimilar methodology now known or hereafter developed.

The use of general descriptive names, registered names, trademarks, service marks, etc. in this publication does not imply, even in the absence of a specific statement, that such names are exempt from the relevant protective laws and regulations and therefore free for general use.

The publisher, the authors, and the editors are safe to assume that the advice and information in this book are believed to be true and accurate at the date of publication. Neither the publisher nor the authors or the editors give a warranty, expressed or implied, with respect to the material contained herein or for any errors or omissions that may have been made. The publisher remains neutral with regard to jurisdictional claims in published maps and institutional affiliations.

This Springer imprint is published by the registered company Springer Nature Switzerland AG
The registered company address is: Gewerbestrasse 11, 6330 Cham, Switzerland

To my parents, Ko-En and Linda, for teaching me that "with diligence, nothing in the world is too difficult," with much love and appreciation.
—David T. Huang

To Tyanna, Sophie, Lily, Jack, and Ethan, whose love makes every day better.
—Travis Prinzi

Book Introduction

In our first edition, we set out to produce an accessible EP book, informed by the experience of attending physicians, the learning process of EP fellows, and the day-to-day practical needs of EP nurses and technologists. In order to accomplish this, the book was edited by the Chief Electrophysiologist at the University of Rochester Medical Center (David Huang, MD) and the Lead EP Technologist (Travis Prinzi, MA, MS, CEPS) at the same institution. Contributions were made both by attending physicians and EP Fellows working in the lab and clinic at that time.

In this new, revised edition, we've continued in that same model, but we have broadened our approach to include the clinical perspective of one of our Nurse Practitioners, Sonja Kreckel, MS, RN, NP-C, CCDS. Most significantly, this contribution will be seen in the added discussion on various means of ambulatory cardiac monitoring, an aspect of EP that has grown tremendously since the first edition.

While the foundational basics of EP remain the same, the technology to assess and treat cardiac arrhythmias has moved along at a rapid pace, resulting in new understandings of arrhythmia circuits and how to treat them. As of the writing of this book, the EP world is on the cusp of a potentially field-changing development of a new treatment modality in pulsed field ablation. By the time you are reading this book, we will likely already know far more about it than we do at its writing. Herein lies the challenge of producing an EP textbook. The field is advancing quickly. We have provided here a book that focuses on the fundamentals that will serve as an important learning tool for us all as students of cardiac electrophysiology in labs and classrooms. We have also pointed to advancing technology and promising developments on the horizon wherever possible.

We also like to pay tribute to all the teachers, both personal and virtual, who have pioneered and advanced the care of patients with cardiac dysrhythmia to where it is today. Specifically, we would mention and remember Drs Mark E Josephson, Hein Wellens, and Arthur Moss for their boundless contributions. Herein we also impart our own advice to all readers to never stop learning while remembering the fundamentals in electrophysiology. We are all fortunate to be involved in a medical field that has continued to advance rapidly.

Contents

1. **Cardiac Conduction and Bradycardia** 1
   Mehmet K. Aktas

2. **Ambulatory Cardiac Rhythm Monitoring** 15
   James Gallagher and Sonja Kreckel

3. **Syncope, Tilt Table Testing, and Cardioversion** 31
   Sarah Taylor

4. **Implantable Cardiac Devices** 47
   Parag Patel, Erin Armenia, and Pina Spampanato

5. **Diagnosis and Treatment of Supraventricular Tachycardias** 81
   Spencer Rosero and Travis Prinzi

6. **Wolff-Parkinson-White (WPW) Syndrome** 103
   Jeffrey M. Vinocur

7. **Atrial Flutter, Typical and Atypical** 129
   David T. Huang and Travis Prinzi

8. **A Practical Guide to Catheter Ablation of Atrial Fibrillation** 147
   Joshua Haswell, Travis Prinzi, and Burr Hall

9 Ventricular Tachyarrhythmias................... 179
Amole Ojo, Sinan Tankut, Travis Prinzi,
and David T. Huang

10 Hereditary Arrhythmias...................... 219
Ido Goldenberg, Alon Barsheshet,
and David T. Huang

Index.. 255

Cardiac Conduction and Bradycardia

Mehmet K. Aktas

Abstract

Bradycardia may be physiological or pathological depending on the underlying mechanism. An understanding of cardiac impulse formation and propagation can help provide insight in differentiating between bradycardia that is benign and those that are pathologic and may require implant of a permanent pacemaker. Patients with bradycardia may present with a wide range of symptoms including shortness of breath, activity intolerance, fatigue, dizziness, presyncope and/or syncope. In some patients, an electrocardiogram (ECG) and external ambulatory heart rhythm monitors are sufficient to document pathological bradycardia. In other instances, patients may require an insertable cardiac monitor, which can provide long-term heart rhythm monitoring. Less often, a patient may require an electrophysiology (EP) study to assess for conduction disease. In this chapter we review common clinical presentations of bradycardia and discuss the diagnostic work up of such patients.

M. K. Aktas (✉)
University of Rochester Medical Center, Rochester, NY, USA
e-mail: mehmet_aktas@urmc.Rochester.edu

© The Author(s), under exclusive license to Springer Nature Switzerland AG 2023
D. T. Huang et al. (eds.), *Cardiac Electrophysiology in Clinical Practice*, In Clinical Practice,
https://doi.org/10.1007/978-3-031-41479-4_1

Keywords

Cardiac conduction · Bradycardia · Sinus node · AV node · His bundle · Heart block · Cardiac anatomy · Electrocardiogram

Sinus Node, Atrioventricular Node, His-Purkinje System

The normal cardiac impulse originates from the sinus node which is a small spindle-shaped structure located anteriorly in the subepicardial region near the junction of the superior vena cava and the right atrium [1]. Normal sinus rhythm (NSR) on an ECG represents normal activation of the heart initiating from the sinus node and activating the rest of the atria and ventricles. Figure 1.1 shows a 3-dimensional electroanatomic map of the right atrium during normal sinus rhythm. The impulse initiated by the sinus node travels through the right atrium and propagates toward the left atrium and simultaneously inferiorly to the atrioventricular (AV) node. The sinus node is innervated by both sympathetic and parasympathetic fibers that modulate the heart rate accordingly [2].

The AV node is located at the apex of the triangle of Koch, which is represented by the septal tricuspid valve annulus anteriorly, the coronary sinus ostium posteriorly, and the tendon of Todaro superiorly [3]. Acting as a gateway, the AV node exhibits decremental properties, whereby rapid stimulation of the AV node results in progressive slowing of conduction, which helps protect the ventricles from tachyarrhythmias starting from the atria which could otherwise result in rapid ventricular rates [4]. From here propagation continues inferiorly and anteriorly to the bundle of His also known as the bundle of Tawara [5]. Once the depolarizing wavefront exits the His bundle, the signal divides into the right (activation the right ventricle) and left (activating the left ventricle) bundle branches of the conduction system. The left bundle further subdivides into the left anterior and left posterior fascicles. Finally, the impulse disseminates throughout the ventricular myocardium via Purkinje fibers.

1 Cardiac Conduction and Bradycardia

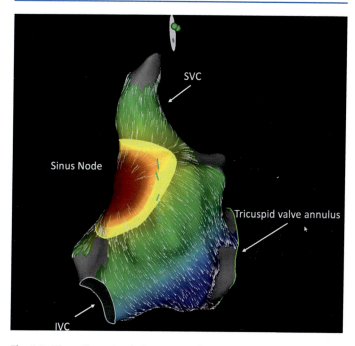

Fig. 1.1 Three-dimensional electroanatomic map of the right atrium during normal sinus rhythm using Carto (Biosense-Webster). Sinus rhythm impulse originates in the high right atrium and propagates throughout the right atrium. Red represents earliest activation which corresponds to the location of the sinus node. Yellow, green, teal, and blue represent respective later activation timing relative to the sinus node impulse. SVC = superior vena cava; IVC = inferior vena cava

Patients may present in NSR with some clues to the presence of conduction disease on the surface ECG which may include either a prolonged PR interval, left anterior fascicular block (LAFB), left posterior fascicular block (LPFB), right bundle branch block (RBBB) or left bundle branch block (LBBB). Some patients may have more than one type of block such as first-degree AV block (defined as a PR > 0.2 s), fascicular block (either left anterior or left posterior), and RBBB; although the term trifascicular block is used to describe this condition, it is incorrect, since the first-degree AV block does occur in a true fascicle but rather represents slow conduction within the atria or AV node.

In patients with LBBB (both left anterior and posterior fascicles are blocked) the conduction to the ventricle occurs through the right bundle branches. Usually the remaining bundle's conduction velocity is adequate to prevent symptoms. However, one should be more suspicious of a bradyarrhythmia as an etiology of symptoms if multiple levels of conduction block are observed on the ECG. Of particular concern is an ECG pattern of alternating RBBB and LBBB, as this is clear evidence of infra-nodal conduction disease. These patients should undergo pacemaker placement without the need for invasive electrophysiology testing as they are at high risk for the development of complete heart block [6].

Each region of cardiac tissue has automaticity, meaning it is capable of spontaneously generating an impulse [7]. However, automaticity within the sinus node establishes a hierarchy of pacemaker function whereby the spontaneous discharge rate of the sinus node exceeds the spontaneous discharge rate of other automatic sites, rendering these sites depressed and latent. When there is failure of impulse generation within the atria, AV nodal automaticity is no longer suppressed, and a junctional rhythm, usually narrow complex, with a rate of 30–40 bpm is observed. If automaticity within the AV junction fails, latent Purkinje fibers may initiate spontaneous depolarizations with slow ventricular rates ranging from 20–30 bpm, with a wide QRS complex.

Sinus Node Dysfunction

Sinus node dysfunction (previously referred to as sick sinus syndrome) is an umbrella term that refers to abnormalities in impulse formation and propagation and includes conditions such as sinus bradycardia, sinus pause/arrest, chronotropic incompetence, sinus exit block, and tachy-brady syndrome where rapid periods of atrial fibrillation terminate often into symptomatic episodes of sinus bradycardia or sinus pauses [8]. Sinus node dysfunction is usually a disease of the elderly and its initial presentation may include syncope due to inadequate impulse formation and propagation, resulting in cerebral hypoperfusion and collapse. Sinus node dysfunction is the most common diagnosis in patients requiring permanent pacemaker implant [9].

The action potentials of both the sinus and AV node are dependent on sodium "funny" currents [10]. These channels are recognized as funny because they open as the cell repolarizes rather than reaching a more positive threshold to evoke an action potential. The sinus node traditionally depolarizes and repolarizes most rapidly and therefore is responsible for setting the heart rate in the normal heart. Sympathetic (adrenaline) and parasympathetic (vagal) signals from the autonomic nervous system have strong influences on heart rate due to their primary inputs to the sinus and AV node. Historically, a "normal" heart rate ranges from 60–100 beats per minute (bpm); however, it is not uncommon for those with high vagal tone (well-conditioned athletes, or during sleep) to have rates as low as 40 bpm [11]. Electrocardiograms may show sinus bradycardia or a junctional escape rhythm (an impulse originating from the AV node). Bradycardia in and of itself is not problematic unless it is associated with symptoms such as dizziness, fatigue, shortness of breath, chest pain, or syncope. Placing these patients on a treadmill may reveal chronotropic incompetence, which refers to the inability of the sinus node to increase the heart rate appropriately with activity. It is important to make the distinction between physiologic bradycardia and symptomatic pathologic bradycardia to avoid unnecessary testing or treatments which may only cause harm and or provide little to no benefit. Furthermore, the etiology of the arrhythmia must strongly be considered. Electrolyte imbalances, ischemia, infection, hypoxia, vagal tone, hypothermia, hypothyroidism, post-surgical state, as well as other causes may be transient, and treating the underlying cause may very well resolve the cardiac conduction disturbance. Temporary pacemakers may be considered in specific emergent situations as deemed necessary.

Atrioventricular Conduction Block

AV block can be classified as first, second, or third degree (also known as complete heart block). Although a distinct conduction fiber or fascicle between the sinus nodeand this His-bundle does not exist, first degree AV block refers to a PR interval exceeding

0.2 s. A long PR interval in the setting of a normal QRS duration usually represents conduction delay within the AV node. If the QRS duration is prolonged, the most common site of conduction delay is still in the AV node; however, the possibility of infra-Hisian conduction disease needs to be considered, especially in the presence of left bundle branch block. It is important to recognize that a normal PR interval does not itself rule out the possibility of more advanced conduction disease. In general, first-degree AV block is clinically well-tolerated and is not associated with an increase in overall mortality. However, in rare cases a PR interval exceeding 0.3 s can produce pacemaker syndrome-like symptoms, where atrial activation begins as ventricular systole continues, and atrial contraction occurs across closed atrio-ventricular valves.

Second degree AV block is subdivided into Mobitz Type 1 and Mobitz Type 2 block. Electrocardiographically, Mobitz type 1 exhibits the Wenckebach phenomenon where progressive prolongation in the PR interval is seen leading up to a non-conducted P wave. Following the non-conducted beat, conduction with a normal PR interval is usually seen. The block cycle recurs repetitively with a fixed P to QRS ratio. Typically there is evidence of grouped beating and periodicity in the conduction pattern observed on the ECG. For example, when 3 P waves results in 2 QRS complexes this is referred to as a 3:2 Wenckebach conduction pattern. This type of block is considered physiological and not pathologic and conduction block typically occurs within the AV node. Mobitz Type 1 block is common in healthy individuals and in states of high vagal innervation such as during sleep. Second degree Mobitz 1 heart block does not require treatment with a pacemaker.

On the other hand, Mobitz Type 2 block demonstrates a fixed PR interval with a non-conducted P wave. On the ECG, the non-conducted P waves are not preceded by prolongation in the PR interval and there is no shortening of the PR interval subsequent to the blocked P wave. In Mobitz Type 2 the block occurs inferior to the His bundle. Second degree Mobitz Type 2 heart block is a pathologic finding and requires further investigation since such patients are at risk for progression to complete heart block. In patients with 2:1 AV nodal conduction as shown in Fig. 1.2, maneuvers like carotid sinus massage, which increases vagal tone, can be useful for differentiating between Mobitz Type 1 and Type 2 block [12]. In Mobitz Type 1 block, higher vagal input to the AV node will increase the amount of blocked p waves. However, in Mobitz Type 2 block, higher vagal input slows the sinus rate which provides the diseased infra-Hisian tissue time to recover allowing for a 1:1 AV nodal conduction (Fig. 1.3).

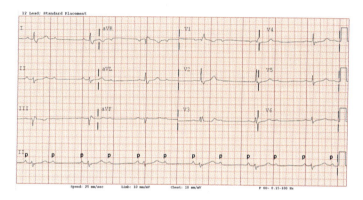

Fig. 1.2 12 lead electrocardiogram demonstrating 2:1 AV block. There are 2 p waves for every QRS complex as seen on the lead II rhythm strip. It is not possible to tell where the level of block is without provocative maneuvers such as having the patient ambulate, vagal maneuvers or administering medications which can inhibit or enhance AV node conduction

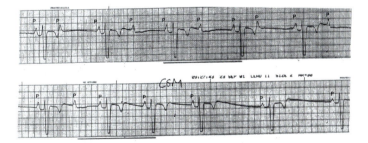

Fig. 1.3 2:1 AV block is present throughout the top telemetry strip. During carotid sinus massage the increased vagal tone results in slowing of the sinus node allowing for 1:1 AV nodal conduction. This is indicative of infranodal disease and best treated with a permanent pacemaker

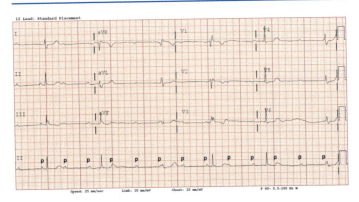

Fig. 1.4 12 lead electrocardiogram demonstrating complete heart block. There are p waves that march through, seen on the rhythm strip lead II with a slow escape rhythm. The site of the escape rhythm appears to change as seen on the rhythm strip

Complete heart block (CHB) is present when atrial activation does not conduct to the ventricles as seen in Fig. 1.4. Complete heart block may occur as a result of pathology within the AV node or in infra-nodal conducting fibers. In patients with CHB often an escape rhythm is present, either a narrow complex junctional rhythm or a wide complex ventricular rhythm. Isorhythmic AV dissociation may make the diagnosis of CHB more difficult as both the atria and ventricles are conducting at the same rate. However, with prolonged heart rhythm monitoring or with exercise testing the presence of atrial and ventricular dissociation can often be detected. Patients with complete heart block may present with shortness of breath, activity intolerance, weakness, dizziness, presyncope, and syncope. Patients with CHB are also at risk for ventricular tachycardia and ventricular fibrillation and therefore require prompt attention and treatment [13].

Electrophysiologic Testing

In some situations, it may be difficult to determine if a patient's symptoms are related to a bradyarrhythmia through non-invasive testing, and an EP study may be required. An EP study allows for an objective measurement of the cardiac conduction system. Catheters are placed into the heart to evaluate for dysfunction of either impulse formation or propagation. Following percutaneous venous access, catheters are typically advanced to the right atrium, the coronary sinus, the bundle of His, and into the right ventricle. These catheters have the ability to both sense electrical potentials and pace. Spanning the catheters into each of the locations facilitates accurate diagnosis and location of potential conduction disease. Baseline measurements which are noted on the surface ECG are recorded, including the PR interval, QRS duration, and QT interval. The intracardiac catheters provide electrograms that correspond to the ECG recordings. The PR interval is represented by the activation from the atria (A) to the His bundle (H) and the ventricular (V) signal. Of particular importance is the assessment of the HV interval. An HV measurement greater than 100 msec is highly abnormal and may warrant pacemaker placement.

Pacing maneuvers during an EP study also provides an objective measurement of the sinus and AV node (both antegrade and retrograde) function. Sinus node recovery time (SNRT) is measured by pacing the atrium for 30 s at a rate faster than the intrinsic sinus rate to suppress sinus node automaticity [14]. The recovery time is measured from the last pacing stimulus to the onset of sinus node activity as recorded on the intra-cardiac electrogram. A SNRT that is less than 1500 milliseconds (msec) is considered normal or less than 550 msec for the corrected SNRT (SNRT minus the sinus cycle length in msec). Patients may also demonstrate sinus node exit block where an electrical impulse is unable to penetrate through the perinodal tissue due to prolonged refractory periods. This may occur either as a Mobitz 1 or 2 block. One may see a sinus rate at 600 ms and then the absence of a p wave at half the interval between the two conducted p waves. The remainder of the sinus rhythm will be consistent at 600 ms.

One can then assess the functional properties of the AV node via pacing stimuli including the cycle length at which Wenckebach occurs or when atrial activation blocks in the AV node and does not conduct into the His bundle. If the block occurs after His activation, then Mobitz Type 2 block is present, which is an important distinction from Wenckebach (Fig. 1.5). During atrial extra-

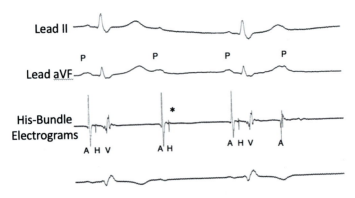

Fig. 1.5 The first sinus beat (labeled A on the His-bundle intracardiac electrograms) conducts through the AV node with subsequent activation of the His bundle (labeled H on the His-bundle electrogram) followed by ventricular activation (labeled V on the His-bundle electrogram). The second sinus beat conducts through the AV node to the His bundle and blocks below the His as denoted by * on the His-bundle recording. The third sinus beat conducts similar to the first beat (A-H-V seen on His-bundle recordings) since the infra-Hisian level of block had time to recover from the prior blocked beat. The last beat is a premature atrial contraction and blocks in the AV node as there is no His activation observed on the His-bundle recording. The second beat is considered pathological and warrants placement of a pacemaker. P = Atrial activation on the surface electrocardiogram. A = atrial activation on the intracardiac electrogram. H=His bundle activation on the intracardiac electrogram. V = ventricular activation on the intracardiac electrogram

stimuli testing, Wenckebach will show AH interval prolongation on the His catheter as the progressively earlier atrial premature beats are delivered. A thorough EPS will help rule out all potential arrhythmogenic etiologies for a patient's clinical presentation. Ventricular pacing can assess the presence of VA or retrograde conduction. Activation should be concentric in the coronary sinus catheter, activating proximally to distally. An eccentric activation sequence can suggest an accessory pathway that may only conduct retrogradely. Understanding the normal functioning properties of the AV node is essential to help exclude the potential for either brady- or tachyarrhythmias.

Concealed Conduction & Incomplete Impulse Penetration

Concealed conduction refers to incomplete impulse penetration into the normal AV nodal conduction system producing ECG findings that could otherwise not be explained, hence the term concealed conduction [15]. Antegrade as well as retrograde concealed conduction into the normal AV nodal conduction system may occur. A common site of retrograde concealment is when a PVC conducts retrogradely into the His-Purkinje system causing antegrade AV block of the following sinus beat.

Gap Phenomenon

A gap in AV conduction is observed when AV conduction block is observed with a premature atrial beat, but a subsequent atrial beat of greater prematurity successfully conducts to the ventricles [16]. The Gap phenomenon occurs as a result of functional differences in conduction present in different regions of the conduction system, often requiring a distal segment with a long refractory period and proximal segment with a shorter refractory period. As such, a premature beat conducts successfully to the distal segment where block occurs. However, with increasing prematurity the beat encounters delayed conduction in the proximal segment giving the distal segment time to recover thereby allowing conduction.

Congenital Heart Block

Newborns may present with conduction disease spanning from first degree block to complete heart block [16]. Children from mothers who have systemic lupus erythematosus are at higher risk of acquiring complete heart block [17]. Antibodies cross the placenta in utero and evoke an immune response that leads to scarring and fibrosis around the AV node. Some patients may have congenital cardiac structural anomalies which may require surgery. In these instances patients may acquire cardiac conduction disease due to post-surgical changes [18].

Neuromuscular Diseases

Clinicians need to be aware of several neuromuscular conditions which are associated with AV block. Common neuromuscular conditions that are associated with cardiac conduction disease include progressive familial heart block, facioscapulohumeral syndrome, myotonic dystrophy, Kearns-Sayre Syndrome, Friedreich's ataxia, and Erb's dystrophy [19, 20]. Progression from normal conduction to high degree AV block may occur rapidly and unpredictably in such patients and therefore close surveillance is recommended.

References

1. Anderson KR, Ho SY, Anderson RH. Location and vascular supply of sinus node in human heart. Br Heart J. 1979;41:28–32.
2. Hanna P, Dacey MJ, Brennan J, Moss A, Robbins S, Achanta S, Biscola NP, Swid MA, Rajendran PS, Mori S, Hadaya JE, Smith EH, Peirce SG, Chen J, Havton LA, Cheng Z, Vadigepalli R, Schwaber J, Lux RL, Efimov I, Tompkins JD, Hoover DB, Ardell JL, Shivkumar K. Innervation and neuronal control of the mammalian sinoatrial node a comprehensive atlas. Circ Res. 2021;128:1279–96.
3. Koch W. Welche Bedeutung kommt dem Sinusknoten zu. Med Klin. 1911;7:447–52.
4. Mani BC, Pavri BB. Dual atrioventricular nodal pathways physiology: a review of relevant anatomy, electrophysiology, and electrocardiographic manifestations. Indian Pacing Electrophysiol J. 2014;14:12–25.
5. Tawara S, Aschoff L. The Conduction System of the Mammalian Heart: Published by Imperial College Press and Distributed by World Scientific Publishing Co.; 2000. ISBN 1-86094-116-8.
6. Bhatt A, Rao S, Infeld M, Greene S, Ambrosy A, Daubert J. Alternating bundle branch block: clinical considerations. J Am Coll Cardiol. 2017;69:2330.
7. Antzelevitch C, Burashnikov A. Overview of basic mechanisms of cardiac arrhythmia. Card Electrophysiol Clin. 2011;3:23–45.

8. Hawks MK, Paul MLB, Malu OO. Sinus node dysfunction. Am Fam Physician. 2021;104:179–85.
9. Adán V, Crown LA. Diagnosis and treatment of sick sinus syndrome. Am Fam Physician. 2003;67:1725–32.
10. DiFrancesco D. The role of the funny current in pacemaker activity. Circ Res. 2010;106:434–46.
11. D'Souza A, Sharma S, Boyett MR. CrossTalk opposing view: bradycardia in the trained athlete is attributable to a downregulation of a pacemaker channel in the sinus node. J Physiol. 2015;593:1749–51.
12. Mangiardi LM, Bonamini R, Conte M, Gaita F, Orzan F, Presbitero P, Brusca A. Bedside evaluation of atrioventricular block with narrow QRS complexes: usefulness of carotid sinus massage and atropine administration. Am J Cardiol. 1982;49:1136–45.
13. Dohadwala M, Kamili F, Estes NMR, Homoud M. Atrioventricular block and pause-dependent torsade de pointes. HeartRhythm Case Rep. 2017;3:115–9.
14. Narula OS, Samet P, Javier RP. Significance of the sinus-node recovery time. Circulation. 1972;45:140–58.
15. Langendorf R, Pick A. Concealed conduction further evaluation of a fundamental aspect of propagation of the cardiac impulse. Circulation. 1956;13:381–99.
16. Wu D, Denes P, Dhingra R, Rosen KM. Nature of the gap phenomenon in man. Circ Res. 1974;34:682–92.
17. Vinet É, Pineau CA, Scott S, Clarke AE, Platt RW, Bernatsky S. Increased congenital heart defects in children born to women with systemic lupus erythematosus. Circulation. 2015;131:149–56.
18. Liberman L, Pass RH, Hordof AJ, Spotnitz HM. Late onset of heart block after open heart surgery for congenital heart disease. Pediatr Cardiol. 2008;29:56–9.
19. Feingold B, Mahle WT, Auerbach S, Clemens P, Domenighetti AA, Jefferies JL, Judge DP, Lal AK, Markham LW, Parks WJ, Tsuda T, Wang PJ, Yoo S-J. Management of Cardiac Involvement Associated with Neuromuscular Diseases: a scientific statement from the American Heart Association. Circulation. 2017;136:e200–31.
20. Bouhouch R, Elhouari T, Oukerraj L, Fellat I, Zarzur J, Bennani R, Arharbi M. Management of cardiac involvement in neuromuscular diseases: review. Open Cardiovasc Med J. 2008;2:93–6.

Ambulatory Cardiac Rhythm Monitoring

James Gallagher and Sonja Kreckel

Abstract

Palpitations and syncope are common symptoms patients report to their healthcare providers that can have significant dysrhythmias associated with them. Some dysrhythmias may lead to sudden death making early identification a priority to determine diagnosis and implement medical/surgical intervention that can be lifesaving. Frequent symptoms are easily assessed via in-office technology such as ECG and Holter. Challenges exist when symptoms are not present at times of evaluation and happen infrequently. Technology has advanced in the field of medical monitoring to include external long term Holters and event monitors as well as real time 30-day continuous monitoring and implantable cardiac monitors. Moreover, patients now have the option to purchase commercially available smartwatch and app ecg systems for their own viewing and can furthermore submit tracings to their health portals for provider review.

J. Gallagher (✉) · S. Kreckel
University of Rochester Medical Center, Rochester, NY, USA
e-mail: james_gallagher@urmc.Rochester.edu

© The Author(s), under exclusive license to Springer Nature Switzerland AG 2023
D. T. Huang et al. (eds.), *Cardiac Electrophysiology in Clinical Practice*, In Clinical Practice,
https://doi.org/10.1007/978-3-031-41479-4_2

Keywords

Holter monitor · Event monitor · MCOT · Implantable cardiac monitor · Palpitations · Syncope · Atrial fibrillation · Tachycardia Bradycardia · ECG · Smartwatch

We live in the Information Age which impacts us immensely. Whether it is "Googling" an answer, attending "YouTube" university before making a home repair, or using wi-fi cameras to monitor your front door, we are surrounded by technology that enables us to access knowledge, record information, and transfer data quickly, often in a small compact devices, such as a cell phone. Medicine is fortunately no exception to this technological progress, particularly in the areas of arrhythmia diagnosis and treatment.

Arrhythmias are common, with an estimated more two million people in the United States having atrial fibrillation, more than 500,000 people with supraventricular tachycardia, and more than 180,000 episodes of sudden cardiac death each year, the majority of which have a ventricular arrhythmia associated [1–3]. In terms of brady-arrhythmias, nearly 200,000 pacemakers are placed each year in the United States [4]. To make the diagnosis of these arrhythmias, an electrocardiogram (ECG) needs to be performed. However, as these arrhythmias are often not present all of the time, doing an intermittent ECG, such as at an office visit, may not catch these events. It is estimated that some patients with atrial fibrillation will go years before it is finally diagnosed on an ECG. As such, cardiac monitors have been developed to continuously recorded the heart rhythm and either store every heart beat, as in a Holter monitor for future analysis; transfer every heart beat for analysis to an offsite technician in near live time, such as with mobile continuous outpatient telemetry (MCOT); or record events as determined by the device or the patient in an event monitor or implantable loop recorder.

In this chapter, we will review the types of cardiac monitoring available and indications for each device.

Holter Monitoring

Portable cardiac monitoring was first performed by Norman "Jeff" Holter in 1947 when he broadcast a radioelectrocardiogram, with more than 80 pounds of equipment carried on his back to record and transmit his heart rhythm [5]. This has now evolved into devices the size of pagers to record continuous ECG from 2 days to 2 weeks.

In the current era, Holter monitoring (see Fig. 2.1) traditionally consists of a battery powered, digital recording device that has three wires connecting the device to patches on the skin. This type of Holter records 24 to 48 hours of a continuous ECG in three different leads which if the patches are placed appropriately should resemble Einthoven's triangle and yield standard lead 1, lead 2 and lead 3 appearance and be comparable to a typical ECG done

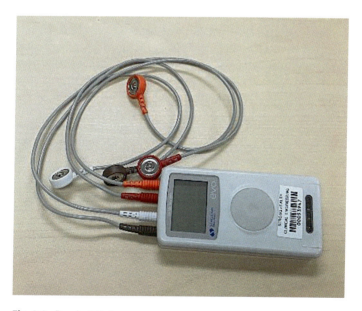

Fig. 2.1 Standard Holter

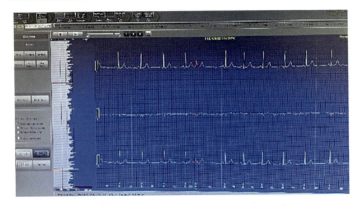

Fig. 2.2 Holter analytic software

in the office. The device is usually not waterproof, and the patient should avoid showering/swimming while wearing. Hypoallergenic patches are available for patients with sensitive skin. If the patient notices palpitations, lightheadedness, near syncope, or other potential cardiac symptoms, they are asked to write down the time so one can correlate the symptom with what rhythm is occurring at that time. After wearing the monitor, the patient turns in the device, and the data is then downloaded and analyzed.

To analyze the data, technicians will use computer software that analyzes not only the rates but each beat's morphology. As the beats are overlayed, abnormal beats are identified and reviewed (Fig. 2.2). The results of this are then compiled into a summary (Fig. 2.3) that typically reports heart rate ranges, frequency of atrial and ventricular ectopy, and sustained arrhythmias and pauses.

Technology continues to progress, and now multiple companies make wearable cardiac monitors that connect to the body with a single patch and a digital recording unit small enough to simply attach to the patch. Data for up to 2 weeks is able to be recorded and the device is waterproof enough that patients can shower with this in place. While there is only one patch, the back of the patch does have multiple electrodes on it, and more than

Holter Summary

Total Beats	232,566	Recording Date	09/13/22
Length Recorded	48 hours 33 minutes	Analysis Date	09/22/22

Overall Rates
Maximum HR 152 bpm on 09/14/22

Mean HR 80 bpm
Minimum HR 56 bpm on 09/14/22 07:53

Ectopy

PVC Beats		PAC Beats	
Count	8	Count	280
Percent	0.00 %	Percent	0.12 %
Max/Hr	3 on 09/14/22 7:0	Max/Hr	44 on 09/13/22 15:0
V-Run	0	SV-Run	1

Pauses 0   Longest on

Ventricular Arrhythmias		Supraventricular Arrhythmias	
VT		SVT	1
Longest	on	Longest	3 on Wed 6:36 AM
Max Rate	on	Max Rate	154 bpm on Wed 6:36 AM
Couplet	1	PAC Couplet	4
Triplet	0	SV-Run	1
R on T			
Bigeminy	0		
Trigeminy	0		
V-Run	0		

Fig. 2.3 Holter report

one "lead" of data can be recorded. The appeal of these patches includes the simplicity of use and up to 2 weeks of continuous recording. Disadvantages are that the data is interpreted by an outside vendor and not all of the data is available for immediate review, but selected episodes chosen by the vendor. Also, morphology of abnormal beats is less distinct, with small vectors between electrodes on the back of the patch compared to typical wider lead placement of a traditional Holter.

Event Monitoring

Event monitors are wireless ambulatory ECG monitors that can record up to a month and are appropriate for aiding in the diagnosis of symptoms that occur infrequently. Event monitors do not have enough storage capacity to record every heartbeat for the whole month, but they can be activated by the user when they feel a symptom and record an ECG of their heart rhythm at that time. In addition, they automatically record when preset heart rate and rhythm criteria have been met (tachycardia above a certain rate, bradycardia below a certain rate, pauses of a certain length or atrial fibrillation, for example). These events are labeled as priority and can result in a phone call from the monitoring company to alert the provider, usually the same day as the event. This is another example of how event monitors differ from Holter monitors; event monitor recordings are interpreted in real time and Holters are reviewed following the completion of testing. The alerts can be adjusted so that one is not called more than they would want, such as having them not alert for a single 2-second pause at night. Of note and something to be explained to patients is that event monitors do not know when the patient is having symptoms. They must be activated to make a recording. There is a built-in diary for patient input of description of the event. An important consideration when choosing an event monitor is to understand that these devices alert for arrhythmias such as atrial fibrillation, but there is no burden data provided, such as percentage of time the patient is in atrial fibrillation. There is no quantification of PVCs or APCs either.

Newer models consist of a small Bluetooth sensor fitted on a patch adhesive that is applied to the upper chest (similar to the newer Holter monitors – see Figs. 2.4 and 2.5). This pairs with a monitor that receives data from the sensor and transmits wirelessly to a data monitoring center. The stored segments are short, lasting between 30-90 seconds. The recording duration of 90 s includes 30 s prior to the event, 30 s during the event and 30 s following the event. Some people have skin sensitivities with the patch, and wearing one for a month is not possible due to skin breakdown or allergy. In this case the sensor may be worn via electrode and single wire electrode.

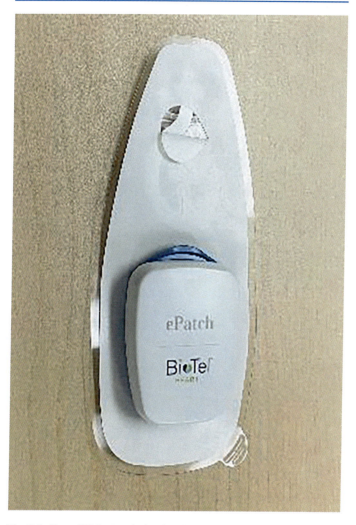

Fig. 2.4 Font of Holter patch showing the recording device attached

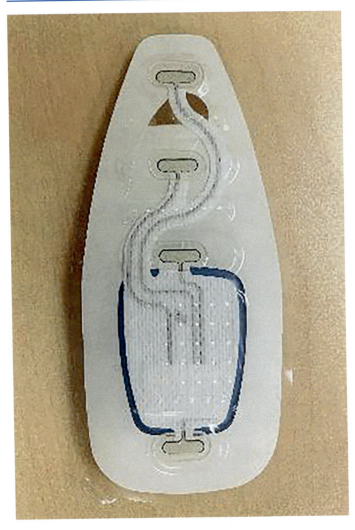

Fig. 2.5 Back of Holter patch showing the electrodes

Mobile Continuous Outpatient Telemetry (MCOT)

Mobile Continuous Outpatient Telemetry (MCOT, Fig. 2.6) is otherwise known as an external cardiac loop recorder. It is a long-term ambulatory ECG monitor with a duration of weeks to one month and is indicated for infrequent cardiac dysrhythmias

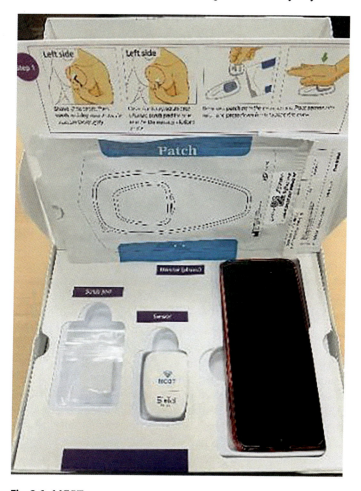

Fig. 2.6 MCOT

associated with concerning symptoms, such as syncope and palpitations. It is similar to the event monitor in that it is a sensor on a patch adhesive that does pre-event recording and post-event recording, as well as auto-triggered events that have met dysrhythmia detection criteria for asystole, bradycardia, tachycardia, and atrial fibrillation. Data is transmitted and interpreted in real time and alert criteria will be followed with a phone call to the provider. The MCOT has additional features that differentiate it from an event monitor, with dysrhythmia detections and heart rate evaluation, p-wave analysis, and QRS morphology analysis. Burden data is provided for AF, PVCs, and APCs. A daily report is submitted to the provider with these analyses, as well as an end of service summary. It is important to note that if an MCOT is not available or declined, downgrading to an event monitor may be acceptable, however the provider must understand that there will be no quantification of AF or ectopic beats (PVCs/APCs).

Implantable Cardiac Monitor (ICM)

An ICM (see Fig. 2.7) is a long-term monitor used for symptoms occurring a few times a year, often when a 30-day event monitor or MCOT has been ineffective because symptoms were not present during the time frame it was worn. The longevity of ICMs is approximately 3 years or more. A common indication for placement of one of these is cryptogenic stroke, looking for silent atrial fibrillation, or with syncope and heightened concern for arrhythmia etiology. The ICM is a monitoring device approximately the size of a large paper clip that is injected under the skin of the chest. It continuously monitors the heart rhythm and records ECG tracings associated with preset detections for asystole, bradycardia, tachycardia, and atrial fibrillation. It provides data on burden of atrial fibrillation, average heart rates both in normal rhythm and when out of rhythm, a comparison of day versus night heart rates, ventricular rate histograms, and correlating activity levels (Fig. 2.8). The ICM can be activated when the patient wants to record an ECG at the time of a symptom. The device recording includes the ECG before the event, through the event, and several minutes after the event

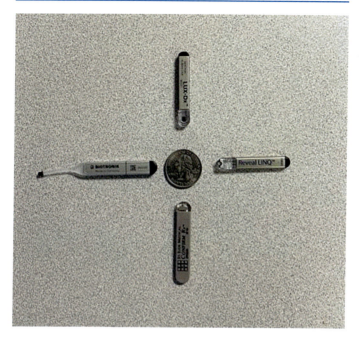

Fig. 2.7 Loop recorders from the four companies that manufacture these: Abbott, Biotronik, Boston Scientific, Medtronic. Size in reference to a quarter

(Fig. 2.9). For example, a nominal setting may be 5.5 minutes pre-event, that gives the patient time to access the recorder activator and then an additional 2.5 minutes following the event. The duration of recording time can be programmed in clinic, knowing the longer one decides to record an event, the fewer events the device can store. Some provide a total of 15 minutes pre- and post-symptom activation, but this allows storage for only two recordings as opposed to four recordings.

The ICM is connected via Bluetooth with a monitor that transmits wirelessly to a database accessed by the provider monitoring the ICM. Newer technologies use a smartphone app monitor, and the advantage to this is the symptom recordings are automatically transmitted within an hour of the symptom event. This eliminates the need to send a manual event to clear storage to make room for more events. Newer ICM models incorporate artificial intelli-

26 J. Gallagher and S. Kreckel

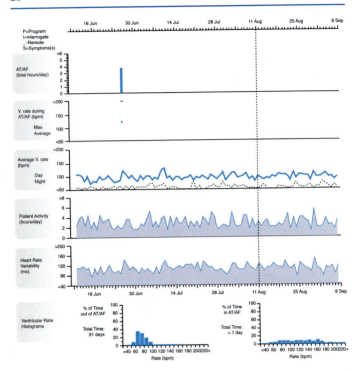

Fig. 2.8 Example loop recorder report

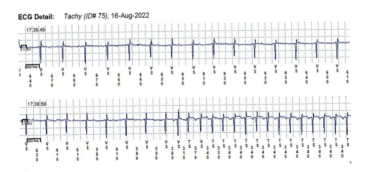

Fig. 2.9 Loop recorder ECG showing onset of SVT

gence (AI) to minimize false positives such as overcalling atrial fibrillation due to oversensing and overcalling pauses due to under detection of QRS complexes.

Over the Counter Home Monitoring Systems

There are a number of home ECG systems that are available, two of which are presently the most dominant on the market: the Apple watch and AliveCor. These systems have led to the democratization of arrhythmia collection, and as a result have patients making their own ECG recordings frequently.

The Apple Watch Series 4 and later models have the ability to perform an ECG by using conductive material on the portion of the watch that rests against the skin and an electrode on the crown of the device which, when touched with the opposite hand, completes a circuit and produces a single lead ECG. This is an ideal way to monitor the heart rhythm, as it can be done any time one is wearing this device. Results the watch may report are sinus rhythm, atrial fibrillation, low or high heart rate, or inconclusive. Apple smartwatches have previously been shown to identify atrial fibrillation looking at pulse irregularity alone with a green LED optical heart sensor to detect pulses in blood flow, independent of an ECG [6]. Current trials are ongoing to identify how digital health tools, such as this watch, which now has an ECG capbility, affect patient care. A limitation of this watch is that it is a single lead ECG and is only active when the patient is touching the watch face, and the ECGS are not high resolution, which can limit the assessment of a tachy-arrhythmia beyond rate alone.

AliveCor is a small Bluetooth-enabled device with two electrodes. An ECG is performed when one places two fingers from each hand on one of two electrodes. This links to one's cell phone where an app presents and records the ECG, which can be saved and sent to the healthcare provider as a PDF file. AliveCor can classify this ECG as sinus rhythm, possible atrial fibrillation, tachycardia, bradycardia, or unclassified/unreadable. AliveCor comes in a single lead and six lead version. In a real-world study from 2018, AliveCor reported that in over 5000 ECGs, about 17%

of ECGs were unclassified and 2% unreadable. If the ECG could be assigned a diagnosis, however, the atrial fibrillation sensitivity was 92%, and the negative predictive value for atrial fibrillation was 98% [7]. In the REHEARSE-AF study, using the AliveCor twice a week in patients ≥65 yo with a CHADSVASC score of ≥2 found atrial fibrillation 4 times as often as routine care in this patient population of more than a 1000 patients [8]. In a prospective, observational trial post-atrial fibrillation ablation comparing a Holter monitor to AliveCor recordings, patients were assigned to wear a Holter for 24+ hours at 3, 6, and 12 months post-procedure. At one of these times, patients were provided with an AliveCor and asked for 4 weeks to do a 30 sec ECG recording three times daily and additionally for any symptomatic episodes. The results showed that more atrial fibrillation recurrences were detected by AliveCor than the serial Holters [9]. One take away from these studies is that the more often one looks for an arrhythmia like atrial fibrillation, the more often one will be found. Home monitoring with systems like AliveCor allow this increase in frequency of monitoring.

Overall, these systems appear to be helpful. They allow patients to record rare arrhythmic events, and on occasion allow asymptomatic patients to be diagnosed with an arrhythmia much sooner, such as atrial fibrillation that could result in stroke. Disadvantages to these systems include that they can not go back in time, such as with an event monitor or loop recorder to record an event several minutes prior. An additional consideration is that patients can make many recordings and ask their health care professional to review large bundles of these events. If every patient made regular recordings and asked their healthcare professional to review all of these ECGs, the data would overwhelm the healthcare system. Fortunately, in our experience, the majority of patients who use these systems use them in a reasonable and appropriate manner.

Conclusion

As technology continues to advance, particularly with devices that can record more data and are smaller to use, as well as products that can be bought over the counter, we are becoming better at documenting arrhythmias. This allows more timely identification of arrhythmias so that appropriate therapy can be started sooner, such as anti-coagulation in patients with atrial fibrillation. This technology will continue to develop in the future, and we look forward to being able to identify patients' arrhythmias in an even more expedited manner.

References

1. Khurshid S, Choi SH, Weng LC, et al. Frequency of cardiac rhythm abnormalities in a half million adults. Circ Arrhythm Electrophysiol. 2018;11:e006273.
2. Orejarena LA, Humberto V Jr, DeStefano F, et al. Paroxysmal supraventricular tachycardia in the general population. J Am Coll Cardiol. 1998;31:150–7.
3. Kong MH, Fonarow GC, Peterson ED. Systematic review of the incidence of sudden cardiac death in the United States. J Am Coll Cardiol. 2011;57:794–801.
4. Greenspon AJ, Patel JD, Lau E, et al. Trends in permanent pacemaker implantation in the United States from 1993 to 2009: increasing complexity of patients and procedures. J Am Coll Cardiol. 2012;60:1540–5.
5. Ioannou K, Ignaszewski M, MacDonald I. Ambulatory electrocardiography: the contribution of Norman Jefferis Holter. BC Med J. 2014;56:86–9.
6. Perez MV, Mahaffey KW, Hedlin H. NEJM. 2019;381:1909–17.
7. Selder JL, Breukel L, van Rossum AC, et al. A mobile one-lead ECG device incorporated in a symptom driven remote arrhythmia monitoring program. The first 5,982 Hartwacht ECGs. Neth Heart J. 2019;27:38–45.
8. Halcox JP, Wareham K, Cardew A, et al. Assessment of remote heart rhythm sampling using the AliveCor heart monitor to screen for atrial fibrillation the REHEARSE-AF study. Circulation. 2017;136:1784–94.
9. Hermans A, Gawalko M, Pluymaekers N, et al. Long-term intermittent versus short continuous heart rhythm monitoring for the detection of atrial fibrillation recurrences after catheter ablation. Int J Cardiol. 2021;329:105–12.

Syncope, Tilt Table Testing, and Cardioversion

3

Sarah Taylor

Abstract

Why do people suddenly lose consciousness? When the issue is cardiac, what can be done about it? While "passing out" is something we are all familiar with, from people "swooning" in movies to sudden cardiac death on the sports field, the reasons and seriousness of a syncopal incident range from the easily diagnosable and treatable to the extremely serious, requiring life-saving intervention. This chapter will explore the reasons for cardiac syncope, how causes are diagnosed, and what treatments are currently available based on diagnosis.

Keywords

Syncope · Tilt table testing · Cardioversion · Sudden cardiac death · Cardiac arrest · Reflex syncope · Orthostatic hypotension

S. Taylor (✉)
Rochester Regional Health, Rochester, NY, USA
e-mail: Sarah.Taylor@rochesterregional.org

© The Author(s), under exclusive license to Springer Nature Switzerland AG 2023
D. T. Huang et al. (eds.), *Cardiac Electrophysiology in Clinical Practice*, In Clinical Practice,
https://doi.org/10.1007/978-3-031-41479-4_3

Syncope is a diagnostic and therapeutic challenge affecting an impressive number of patients. Syncope accounts for 3% of emergency room visit and 6% of all hospital admissions [1]. The lifetime incidence of syncope is close to 40% [2]. Syncope has a bimodal distribution of occurrence. The prevalence is high between 10–30 years, not a common occurrence in middle life, and then peaks again after the age of 65.

One of the most interested yet challenging features regarding the management of syncope is the diverse range of significance of a syncopal episode. Syncope can be a very benign, explicable almost anticipated outcome of a predictable setting. On the other hand, syncope may the one and only presenting symptom of a life threatening disease. Given the staggeringly broad causes and consequences of a syncopal episode, the treating physician has two goals.

1. Identify the cause of the syncope in order to guide treatment based on the underlying etiology
2. Identify the specific risk to the patient. This includes not only the risk of recurrent syncope, but also the risks associated with the underlying [3].

For the physician managing syncope, risk stratification, which is based on the etiology of the syncopal episode, becomes perhaps the most important role.

Syncope is derived from the Greek word synkopē, which means "to cut short" or "to interrupt". Syncope is defined by transient loss of consciousness due to global cerebral hypoperfusion. Syncope is characterized by rapid onset, short duration, and spontaneous complete recovery.

There are many syndromes that may present as masquerading syncope. These include falls, cataplexy, TIAs, seizures, psychogenic pseudosyncope, metabolic disorders, intoxication, and vertebrobasilar insufficiency. Because of confusion in the etiology of these episodes, many of these patients are referred to the electrophysiologist for the evaluation of the cardiac conduction system. It is important to discern the features that suggest a non-syncopal alternation in consciousness. A thorough history should differentiate these other forms of altered consciousness from the sudden loss of consciousness due to a global, reversible reduction in blood flow.

Testing done in the electrophysiology lab is performed to evaluate whether syncope resulted from bradycardia, tachycardia, or a reproducible cardiac reflex or autonomic abnormality. Prior to undergoing testing, a thorough history is essential to help correctly classify syncope. The 2009 European Society of Cardiology guidelines for the management of syncope provide an excellent framework for the classification of syncope based on etiology.

Insufficient cerebral perfusion is the hallmark of syncope. The insults that result in an abrupt reduction of cerebral blood flow are many and varied. A fall in systemic blood pressure curtails global cerebral blood flow. If blood flow is significant diminished for as short as for 6–8 s, syncope may ensue. Systemic blood pressure is determined by systemic vascular resistance and cardiac output. Cardiac output is the product of heart rate and stroke volume. Syncope may result from a decrease in peripheral vascular resistance, a reduction in heart rate, a reduction in stroke volume, or a reduction in a combination of mechanisms (see Fig. 3.1 for incidence).

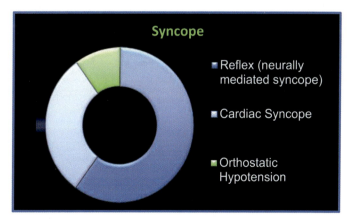

Fig. 3.1 Relative Incidence of syncope by pathophysiological classification

Reflex Syncope

Reflex syncope (see Fig. 3.2 for summary), also correctly termed neutrally mediated syncope, accounts for more than half of syncope. Determining the mechanism of the reflex syncope episodes is paramount for effective treatment and prevention. Reflex syncope should be thought of as a spectrum of inappropriate reflexes. Vasodepressor syncope, characterized by a profound hypotensive response is at one end of the spectrum and cardioinhibitory

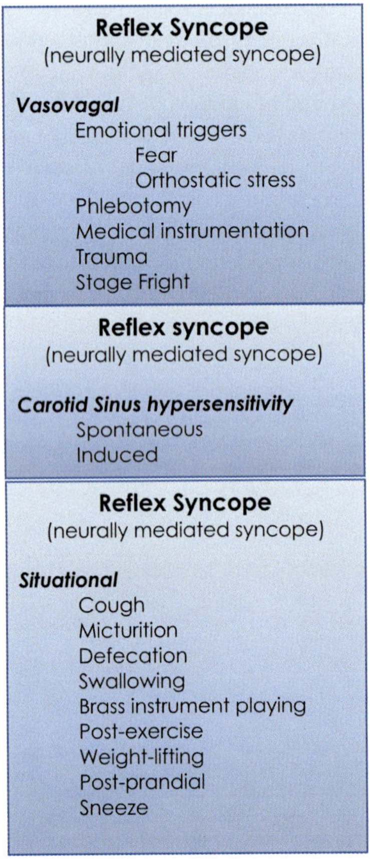

Fig. 3.2 Summary of reflex syncope

Reflex Syncope
(neurally mediated syncope)

Vasovagal
- Emotional triggers
  - Fear
  - Orthostatic stress
- Phlebotomy
- Medical instrumentation
- Trauma
- Stage Fright

Reflex syncope
(neurally mediated syncope)

Carotid Sinus hypersensitivity
- Spontaneous
- Induced

Reflex Syncope
(neurally mediated syncope)

Situational
- Cough
- Micturition
- Defecation
- Swallowing
- Brass instrument playing
- Post-exercise
- Weight-lifting
- Post-prandial
- Sneeze

syncope, characterized by asystolic pauses, is at the other end of the spectrum. While the etiology is the same, the hemodynamic responses may be markedly different. Identifying where on this spectrum the patient lies, guides the treating physician to effective therapy. No longer is it appropriate to apply across the board treatment to the spectrum of neutrally mediated syncope. For patients in whom a vasodepressor response is the overriding perturbation, volume expansion, vasoconstriction and blood pressure augmentation is the mainstay of treatment. Patients that have a primary cardioinhibitory response to reflex-provoking stimuli may benefit from pacemaker therapy. This has been demonstrated in the Eastbourne Syncope Assessment Study, where implantable loop recorders effectively guided syncope therapy [4].

The most common etiology of syncope is a neutrally mediated reflex triggered by different stimuli leading to sudden withdrawal of sympathetic activity and to an increase in parasympathetic nerve tone. The results are vasodilatation and bradycardia. Neurally mediated syncope is classically precipitated extrinsic factors, be it physical or emotional triggers. This includes prolonged standing leading to venous pooling as well as emotional triggers such as fear, needle phobia, pain, and stage fright.

Another form of neutrally mediated syncope is situational syncope. There are specific triggers that elicit abnormal hemodynamic responses leading to the symptomatic global hypoperfusion.

Carotid sinus hypersensitivity is another form of reflex syncope. While other forms of reflex syncope may occurs throughout all stages of life, this typically presents >50 years of age. It is more common in men than in women. An abnormal response to carotid sinus massage is defined as a pause for more than 3 s or a drop in systolic blood pressure greater than 50 mmHg. Normally a mixed picture of vasodepressor and cardioinhibitory response is elicited.

Syncope Due to Orthostatic Hypotension

An abnormal vasoconstriction response to upright position can results in decreased cerebral perfusion. When upright, 10–15% of blood pools in the lower extremities. The baroreceptors are acti-

Fig. 3.3 Orthostatic hypotension

> **Orthostatic Hypotension**
>
> **Volume depletion**
> Hemorrhage
> Gastrointestinal losses
> **Medication**
> Vasodilators
> Alpha-blockers
> Diuretics
> Neuromodulators
> **Primary autonomic failure**
> Multiple–system atrophy
> Parkinson's
> Pure autonomic failure

vated by the decreased pressure that results from this drop in venous return and drop in stroke volume. A normal response increased heart rate, increased contractility and restored vascular tone. However, an abnormal response to these triggers may result in orthostatic intolerance if normal stroke volume is not restored. An abnormal response to upright posture is defined as a decrease in systolic blood pressure > 20 mmHg or a decrease of symptomatic fall of systolic blood pressure associated with syncope or presyncope. (See Fig. 3.3 for summary.)

Cardiac Syncope

Cardiac syncope (see Fig. 3.4) requires the most accurate diagnosis, as it may be the first sign of a life-threatening disorder. The absence of a prodrome is a common feature of these high-risk syncope scenarios. As a result, the risk of trauma is much higher with cardiac syncope. Exertional syncope should initiate a search for a cardiac cause of syncope.

> *The only difference between syncope and sudden death is that in one you wake up—George Engel*

Cardiac Syncope

Tachyarrhythmia
  Supraventricular tachycardia
  Atrial fibrillation
  AVNRT
  AVRT
  Wolff-Parkinson White syndrome

Ventricular tachyarrhythmias
  Long QT syndrome
  Ischemia
  Hypertrophic Cardiomyopathy
  ARVD
  Short QT syndrome
  Brugada Syndrome
  CPVT
  Cardiac Sarcoidosis
  Drugs
  Idiopathic VF
  Left ventricular dysfunction

Bradyarrhythmia
  Sinus node arrest
  Sinoatrial block
  AV block
    Infrahisian conduction
  disease Pacemaker or ICD
  malfunction

Structural Heart Abnormalities
  Aortic Stenosis
  Hypertrophic Cardiomyopathy
  Mitral Stenosis
  Atrial myxoma
  Pericardial Tamponade
  Pulmonary Hypertension
  Pulmonary Embolism
  Myocardial ischemia or infarction

Fig. 3.4 Cardiac syncope

Obstruction to cardiac output is another cause of syncope. While this type of cardiac syncope is less common, it carries with it a high mortality [5].

Arrhythmias also impede cardiac output. The sudden change in heart rate, wither fast or slow, may drastically reduce the cardiac output. In some patients with SVT, the cardiac output is still sufficient to maintain cerebral perfusion, but a mixed picture with a vasodepressor response occurs, resulting in syncope [6].

In patient with a suspicion for arrhythmogenic syncope but undocumented rhythm disturbances, lengthy monitoring is often required. The implantable loop recorder has proven to be very useful in this regard. The ILR provides a cost-efficient and timely method to correlate heart rhythm at the time of syncope or presyncopal symptoms (see Chap. 2). This leads to the appropriate intervention, be it pacemaker, defibrillator, electrophysiology study with ablation, or medical therapy. Even documenting normal sinus rhythm at the time of symptoms can efficiently reroute the management in the effective direction.

Editor's Note Significant advances recently have been reported in the treatment for neurocardiogenic syncope. The Heart Rhythm Society released a press report during the 2022 Scientific Sessions stating that "Cardioneural ablation could replace need for pacemaker in young patients with vasovagal syncope and episodes of slow heart rate." In the past, patients with profound bradycardia or prolonged pauses may undergo a pacemaker implant as treatment if they experience recurrent symptoms. Long term implanted cardiac devices may have implications of lead fracture, multiple generator changes or even potential infection especially in younger patients. This type of ablation targeting atrial ganglionic plexi may be an effective therapy for patients with either cardio-inhibitory or vasodepressor variants of syncope. Further large scaled randomized trials or a prospective registry are needed to further confirm the results and advance this promising therapeutic procedure.

Tilt Table Testing

Tilt table testing is utilized to help investigate the underlying cause of unexplained syncope. Tilt table testing was first used to diagnose syncope in 1986 [7]. The test helps demonstrate the hemodynamic response to a passive upright challenge. It can help define the mechanism with neutrally mediated syncope or orthostatic hypotension syncope is suspected. If the detailed clinical history, along with a normal exam, normal echo, and normal ECG all suggest neutrally mediated syncope, a tilt table test may not be necessary to solidify the diagnosis [8]. However, there are times when a formal test is useful. Fortunately, tilt table testing is easy, safe, well tolerated, and often contributes to the patients understanding of their clinical situation. It also plays a role in defining dysautonomia syndromes, such as postural orthostatic tachycardia syndrome and orthostatic intolerance.

Tilt table testing is also utilized to diagnose pseudosyncope, recurrent falls, and occasionally for medication guidance. Tilt table testing has been useful for initiating and monitoring pyridostigmine therapy. Tilt table testing with EEG can be useful for differentiating seizures from syncope, as well as for diagnosed pseudoseizures or pseudosyncope. (See Fig. 3.5 for contraindications.)

Tilt table testing can be performed safely at all ages [9, 10]. Well operating equipment is paramount. Attentive staff with con-

Fig. 3.5 Contraindications for tilt testing

Contraindications for tilt testing

Inability to cooperate
Pregnancy
Critical Valvular Stenosis
LVOT obstruction
Severe proximal cerebral stenosis
Severe coronary artery disease
Recent MI
Recent CVA
Weight that exceeds safe table operation

tinuous hemodynamic monitoring is required. The tilt must be able to be reliably and quickly reversed. While there are rare reports of arrhythmias and myocardial infarction during tilt table testing, these risks are typically related to the provocation. There are no reports of death from tilt table testing.

Ideally, tilt table testing should be carried out in a room free of distractions and overstimulation. The environment should be at a constant temperature, avoiding excessing heat or cold to avoid autonomic triggers. The test should be observed continuously as restoring the patient to the supine position is integral to restoring cerebral perfusion.

Protocols to improve the sensitivity of the tilt table test include using provocative agents. Isoproterenol infusions have been used. Nitroglycerin is a provocative agent that is better tolerated, especially in elderly patients [11]. The 'Italian Protocol" for upright tilt test involves a stabilization phase of 5 min in the supine position, passive tilt phase of 20 min at a tilt angle of 60 degrees; and provocation phase of further 15 min of 60° tilt after sublingual nitroglycerin. Carotid sinus massage during tilt can also increase the diagnostic yield of testing for carotid sinus hypersensitivity. Care must be taken to weigh the risk of stroke during carotid massage, as the risk is approximately 1:1000, [12].

The test should be completed to the end of protocol. Test interruption is made when the protocol is completed in the absence of symptoms, or there is occurrence of syncope, or occurrence of progressive (>5 min) orthostatic hypotension [13]. Transient asystole, and at times prolonged asystole, may be precipitated. Rarely are interventions other than returning to supine are required (see Fig. 3.6).

> Reasons for early termination of tilt table testing
>
> Syncope
> Systolic BP < 70mmHg or rapid decline
> Bradycardia <50 bpm or rapid decline
> Excessive tachycardia (exceeding 220-age)
> Significant Arrhythmias
> Hyperventilation leading to ETCO2<20mmHg
> Patient distress
> Unstable patient positioning

Fig. 3.6 Reasons to terminate tilt test

Interpreting the Results

A positive tilt table test demonstrates an abnormal hemodynamic response to upright challenge with the symptom reproduction. When a patient's syncope or presyncope symptoms are reproduced and accompanied by bradycardia and hypotension, a diagnosis of neutrally mediated syncope is suspected. The degree of relative bradycardia versus hypotension can help elucidate cardioinhibitory versus vasodepressor syncope. When hemodynamic changes occur in the absence of symptoms, the test is deemed a false positive. Clearly, a limiting feature of tilt table test is the false positive response to the test. The test must be interpreted in the context of the clinical scenario (Fig. 3.7).

Cardioversion

Perhaps the simplest yet most utilized and useful tool in cardiac electrophysiology is the cardioversion (see Fig. 3.8 for summary). It is also the most historical application of electricity. In fact an animal application in poultry to induce and correct arrhythmias was documented in the eighteenth century [14]. Karl Ludwig applied electrical current to a canine heart in 1850 [15]. The first

> **Hemodynamic Response to Upright Tilt Test**
>
> **Postural Orthostatic Tachycardia Syndrome**
> Heart rate exceeds >130 bpm in the first 10 minutes of upright challenge. Significant hypotension is not part of the typical response.
>
> **Vasodepressor**
> Decline in blood pressure with the absence of heart rate decline >10%
>
> **CardioInhibitory**
> Heart rate drops to <40pm
> Asystolic response
>
> **Mixed Hemodynamic response**
> Bradycardia with hypotension
>
> **Orthostatic Hypotension**
> Sustained fall in systolic blood pressure >20mmHG or diastolic blood pressure >10mmHg in the first 3 minutes of tilt

Cardioversion

Fig. 3.7 Hemodynamic response to tilt test

> **Guide for Successful Cardioversion**
>
> Adequate skin preparation
>
> Dry, clean, and hairless
>
> Optimal electrode placement for optimal current flow
>
> AP placement is preferable
>
> Anterior pad should be on the right lateral border of the sternum centered over the fourth intercostal space.
>
> Posterior pad should be placed adjacent to the left of the spine with the center of the electrode at the level of the T7 vertebra.
>
> No air pockets or uneven adhesion of pads
>
> Appropriate selection of energy
>
> For atrial flutter, energy levels between 30-100 joules biphasic will be effective
>
> For atrial fibrillation, energy levels between 75-200 joules biphasic will be necessary. In a patient with an excessive thoracic diameter, 200-300 joules biphasic may be necessary.

Fig. 3.8 Cardioversion summary

3 Syncope, Tilt Table Testing, and Cardioversion

human intentional application was in 1947 using DC defibrillation during cardiac surgery. The first application of cardioversion to convert atrial fibrillation was in 1962. Lown utilized synchronized DC shocks to restore normal sinus rhythm. (Lown, Defibrillation and cardioversion, [16]) (Lown, Amarasingham, & Neuman, New method for terminating cardiac arrhythmias. Unse of synchronized capacitor discharge, [17]).

More recent improvements in the technique of cardioversion include using defibrillation electrodes or pads that adhere to the patient's skin rather than using paddles. Another advancement that has improved the efficacy of energy delivery to the heart while minimizing concurrent myocardial damage is the use of biphasic rather than monophasic waveforms.

Prior to cardioversion, electrolytes should be evaluated and corrected if abnormal. If necessary, digoxin levels should be evaluated and acute myocardial infarction excluded. Anticoagulation should be administered prior to cardioversion. Documentation of adequate uninterrupted anticoagulation in the weeks prior to cardioversion is necessary to minimize the risk of cardioembolic phenomenon. If adequate anticoagulation cannot be ensured, TEE-guided cardioversion should be employed. While traditionally the duration of AF that mandated anticoagulation was thought to be 48 h, there is increasing data suggesting that the risk of stroke may be associated with much shorter episodes of AF [18, 19].

Adequate monitored anesthesia care or monitored sedation is a critical part of cardioversion. Patient comfort in this elective procedure is paramount. Synchronization of the electrical discharge with the QRS complex is what differentiates cardioversion from defibrillation. By timing the electrical discharge with the QRS, the vulnerable period of the T wave is avoided. The risk of inducing ventricular fibrillation exists is a shock was delivered during this vulnerable window. Defibrillation is an unsynchronized delivery of energy used to convert ventricular fibrillation. Care should be taken not to try to synchronize the defibrillation to a rhythm of ventricular fibrillation as delays in therapy may occur. When an electrical current delivered across the myocardium, the cells are simultaneously depolarized, reset, and permit restoration of sinus node activation. The sinus node takes over as the effective pacemaker. Cardioversion is effective for the termination of atrial fibrillation, ventricular tachycardia, or reentrant SVTs. Some arrhythmias will not terminate with cardioversion, notably arrhythmias due to increased automaticity. This includes digitalis-induced tachycardia, catecholamine induced arrhythmia, and some focal atrial tachycardias.

Once the electrodes and defibrillation pads are applies, the defibrillator should be synchronized to detect the patients R waves. When adequately sedated, the energy level is selected and the shock button is pressed and held until discharge. There is a momentarily delay until the defibrillator discharges with the next detected R wave, thereby avoiding delivering energy in the vulnerable period of the cardiac cycle.

Care should be taken to avoid exposure to high flow oxygen. In an oxygen risk environment, electrical sparking from the paddles could ignite a fire. Fortunately, there are no reports of fires occurring when using the adhesive pads. If first shock is not successful, examine the pads for optimal location and adherence. If necessary, replace pads. Consider repositioning anterior pad to optimize the direction of current flow delivered. With proper technique and safety precautions, cardioversion remains an effective, safe, low risk, economical and well-tolerated procedure [20].

References

1. Sun BC, Emond J. Direct medical costs of synocpe-related hospitalizations in the United States. Am J Cardiol. 2005;95(5):668–71.
2. Ganzeboom KS, Mairuhu G, Reitmas J, Linzer M, Weiling W, van Dijk N. Lifetime cumulative incidence of syncope int the general population: a study of 549 Dutch subjects aged 35-60 years. J Cardiovasc Electrophysiol. 2006;17(11):1172–6.
3. Moya AE. Guidelines for the diagnosis and management of syncope version 2009 n.d..
4. Farwell D, Freemantle N, Sulke N. The clinical impact of implantable loop recorders in patients with syncope. Eur Heart J. 2006;27:351–6.
5. Numeroso, F., Mossini, G., Lippi, G., & Cervellin, G.. Evaluation of the current prognostic role of heart diseases in the history of patients with syncope (2014, January 31).

6. Leitch J, Klein GJ, Yee R, Leather RA, Kim YH. Syncope associated with supraventricular tachycardia. An expression of tachycardia rate or vasomotor response? Circulation. 1992;85:1064–71.
7. Kenny R, Ingram A, Bayliss J, Sutton R. Head-up tilt: a useful test for investigating unexplained syncope. Lancet. 1986;1:1352–5.
8. Brignole M, Alboni P, Benditt D, Bergfeldt L, Blanc J, Bloch Thomsen P, et al. Guidelines on management (diagnosis and treatment) of syncope. Eur Heart J. 2001;22(15):1256–306.
9. Tan M, Parry S. Vasovagal syncope in the older patient. J Am Coll Cardiol. 2008;51:599–606.
10. Gieroba Z, Newton J, Parry S, Norton M, Lawson J, Kenny R. Unprovoked and glyceryl trinitrate-provoked head-up tilt table test is safe in older people: a review of 10 Years' experience. J Am Geriatr Soc. 2004;52(11):1913–5.
11. Timoteo AT, Oliveira MM, Feliciano J, Antunes E, Nogueira da Silva M, Silva S, et al. Head-up tilt testing with different nitroglycerin dosages: experience in elderly patients with unexplained sycnope. Europace. 2008;10(9):1091–4.
12. Richardson D, Bexton R, Shaw F, Steen N, Bond J, Kenny R. Complications of carotid sinus massage—a prospective series of older patients. Age Ageing. 2000;29(5):413–7.
13. Bartoletti A, Alboni P, Ammirati F, Brignole M, Del Rosso A, Foglia Manzillo F, et al. The Italian protocol: a simplified head-up tilt testing potentiated with oral nitroflycerin to assess patients with unexplained syncope. Europace. 2000;2(4):339–42.
14. Abilgard C. Tentamina electica in animalibus institua. Societatis Medicae Hayneiensis Colectanea. 1775;2:157.
15. Roth N. First stammering of the heart: Ludwig's lymograph. Med Instrum. n.d.;12:348.
16. Lown B. Defibrillation and cardioversion. Cardiovasc Res. 2002;55(2):220–4.
17. Lown B, Amarasingham R, Neuman J. New method for terminating cardiac arrhythmias. Unse of synchronized capacitor discharge. JAMA. 1962;182:548–55.
18. Bernstein RA. Cryptogenic stroke and underlying atrial fibrillation n.d..
19. Glotzer T, Daoud E, Wyse D, Singer D, Ezekowitz M, Hilker C, et al. The relationship between daily atrial tachycarrhythmia burden from implantable device diagnostics and stroke risk. The TRENDS STudy. Circ Arrhythm Electrophysiol. 2009;2:474–80.
20. Botkina S, Dhanekulaa L, Olshansky B. Outpatient cardioversion of atrial arrhythmias: efficacy, safety, and costs. Am Heart J. 2003;145(2):233–8.

Implantable Cardiac Devices

4

Parag Patel, Erin Armenia,
and Pina Spampanato

Abstract

Modern device therapy has its roots going back to the 1950s. In the ensuing decades a pacemaker has gone from an external battery-powered device to a fully implantable system. Advent of the fully implantable cardiac defibrillator has been lifesaving for patients with ventricular arrhythmias. Over time these devices have become very sophisticated, evolving from a device that would simply pace the heart to one that is a complex sensor, logbook, battery, and, of course, a life saving device.

Keywords

Pacemaker · Implantable cardiac defibrillator · Defibrillation threshold testing · Cardiac resynchronization therapy · His

P. Patel (✉) · P. Spampanato
Cardiology and Electrophysiology, University of Rochester Medical Center, Rochester, NY, USA
e-mail: Parag_Patel@urmc.Rochester.edu

E. Armenia
Clinical Cardiac Electrophysiology Fellow, University of Rochester Medical Center, Rochester, NY, USA

© The Author(s), under exclusive license to Springer Nature Switzerland AG 2023
D. T. Huang et al. (eds.), *Cardiac Electrophysiology in Clinical Practice*, In Clinical Practice,
https://doi.org/10.1007/978-3-031-41479-4_4

bundle pacing · Left bundle branch pacing · Interrogation · Threshold · Sensing · Impedance

Device-based therapy has now become routine with these innovations benefiting millions of patients. In this chapter we will learn about these devices, which are a cornerstone in the field of cardiac electrophysiology exploring indications, procedural implant, device follow up and emerging technologies.

Indications for Permanent Pacing

The cardiac conduction system consists of the SA node, the AV node, the His bundle, and the bundle branches dividing into the Purkinje system. Irreversible abnormalities at any of these structures causing symptomatic bradycardia are typical indications for permanent pacing.

Sinus node dysfunction, sick sinus syndrome, and chronotropic incompetence are a collection of diseases that are quite common with an increasing incidence related to aging. In patients with symptoms which correlate to sinus node dysfunction, pacing is a Class 1 indication. Symptoms may range from fatigue or exertional limitations to a more dramatic presentation of syncope. Sinus bradycardia may also result from medications which are needed for other diseases, and in these cases pacing may also be required.

Atrioventricular block is another common indication for permanent pacing. In patients with second degree AV block, it is important to differentiate between Mobitz type I and Mobitz type 2 AV block, as it is the latter which requires permanent pacing as opposed to the former; although with the presence of significant symptoms, pacing is an option for the former. Permanent pacing is often required in patients with third degree AV block even in the absence of symptoms. Normal exceptions would include reversible conditions such as Lyme disease or in asymptomatic patients with congenital AV block. For a more comprehensive review, the authors refer the reader to 2018 ACC/AHA/HRS Guideline on the Evaluation and Management of Patients With Bradycardia and Cardiac Conduction Delay: A Report of the American College of Cardiology/American Heart Association Task Force on Clinical Practice Guidelines and the Heart Rhythm Society [1] and the ACC/AHA/HRS Versus ESC Guideline for the Diagnosis and Management of Syncope [2].

A key element in recommending permanent pacing is the presence of symptoms, as often bradycardia is noted in asymptomatic patients. To correlate symptoms, long term holter monitoring and at times implantable loop recorder monitoring may be necessary [3]. A notable exception, however, is the presence of advanced conduction system disease and heart block below the level of the atrioventricular node, as this is usually irreversible with an unpredictable course. The choice of deciding between a single and dual chamber pacemaker depends on the underlying condition. In patients with AV block and preserved sinus node function, a dual chamber device is preferred to maintain atrioventricular synchrony. Additionally, even in patients who have isolated SA node disease, a dual chamber device may be preferred, as they may develop AV block in the future. In patients who require ventricular pacing in the setting of longstanding permanent atrial fibrillation with no plan to restore sinus rhythm, a single ventricular lead is indicated.

Pacemaker System

The pacemaker system consists of a pacemaker pulse generator along with implantable leads. The generator consists of a lithium-iodine battery and a circuitry board. The unit is housed in a hermetically sealed, inert titanium or titanium alloy casing. A polyurethane-based header houses the ports for which the pacing leads are plugged into. The typical battery life of a normally functioning pacemaker ranges from 8 to 15 years depending on many factors such as the size of the battery, percentage of pacing, voltage stimulation required, and chronic impedance.

Device Implantation

Once it has been determined the patient qualifies for a pacemaker, the rationale for the procedure and risks involved are reviewed with the patient. The pacemaker implant procedure is quite safe, with very serious complications on the order of 1% or 2%. Typical procedural risks include pneumothorax, cardiac perforation with tamponade, and excessive bleeding. Attention to sterile preparation and implantation technique is of utmost importance to prevent short to medium term infections. The greater majority of implants are placed in the left upper chest of the patient, as most people are right-handed. However, when required, right-sided implants can be done in a similar fashion.

For patient comfort usually moderate sedation is provided, and then the patient is prepped and draped in a sterile fashion. In most cases an ipsilateral peripheral venogram (Fig. 4.1) is performed for identification of the axillary/subclavian venous system.

This allows for visualization of the venous drainage system into the right heart, any narrowing or obstruction, or in the rare case a left sided SVC. The typical location of the axillary vein is approximately 1 cm below the subclavian vein overlying the first rib. Lidocaine is then infiltrated subcutaneously approximately 2–3 cm below the clavicle and medial to the delta pectoral groove. A 3-to-4-centimeter skin incision is made, and then the subcutaneous fat layer is dissected down to the anterior pectoral fascia with electrocautery. If there is enough subcutaneous tissue, a pocket is fashioned inferomedially along the anterior pectoral fascial plane large enough to hold the device. In patients with minimal subcutaneous tissue the pectoral muscle can be divided to the subpectoral plane, and a pocket can be fashioned to provide better tissue coverage for the implanted device. Next, the axillary vein is accessed via modified Seldinger technique and guide wires are passed into the right heart or inferior vena cava. Confirming venous and not arterial access is essential prior to sheath insertion. It is preferred to access the vein prior to its course under the subclavian vein to avoid an insulation erosion or crush injury via the "nutcracker" phenomena between the lead, first rib, and clavicle

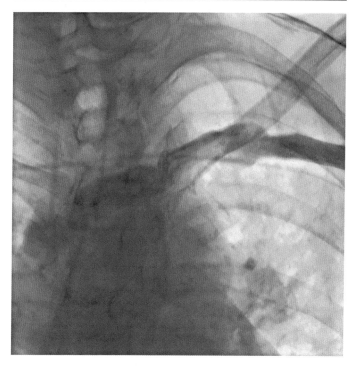

Fig. 4.1 Peripheral venogram

over time. Once successful access is obtained a peelable sheath is advanced over the guidewire into the axillary vein. In a dual chamber system usually the right ventricular lead is placed first. This is performed by shaping the inner stylet so that the lead can initially be advanced into the right ventricular outflow tract. The lead is advanced into the vein and carefully to the right heart with the stylet not fully at the tip initially so that the lead tip is soft. Once the lead is in the right atrium, the pre-shaped stylet is advanced to the tip, and the lead is advanced across the tricuspid valve into the right ventricular outflow tract. The stylet is removed. Next, another stylet is shaped with a 90-degree bend, and this is advanced through the lumen to the lead tip. The lead is then slowly retracted with counterclockwise torque so that the tip points towards the septum. Once the lead drops into the right ventricle, it is advanced towards the mid to distal septum until tissue contact is made. It is preferred to avoid lateral or apical placement to minimize the risk of cardiac perforation. Once the lead is in a suitable location, the active fixation screw is deployed and full deployment is confirmed under fluoroscopy. The stylet is then withdrawn, and the lead is tested in a bipolar fashion for sensing, impedance, and threshold. Tissue injury is also assessed via the local electrogram. Significant tissue injury, R waves greater than 4 millivolts, stable impendence, and initial threshold under 2 V at 0.4 ms are all consistent with acceptable lead placement. Over the ensuing minutes, as tissue injury dissipates, R wave sensing will usually rise, and the pacing threshold will decrease. Sufficient slack is then placed in the lead, and the lead is secured with silk suture to the pectoralis muscle via the suture sleeve.

Following placement of the ventricular lead, the atrial lead is placed. In a similar manner the lead is advanced through a peelable sheath to the mid right atrium. A pre-shaped J curve style is then advanced into the lead which usually will deflect the tip of the lead towards the right atrial appendage. Gentle advancement and retraction can confirm distal fixation of the lead in the appendage. If the site is not adequate, clockwise and counterclockwise movement may be needed to move the lead into the right atrial appendage. Classically, the lead tip will wag like a dog's tail when in the appendage, although this is not always seen. Once the tip is in a desirable location, the active fixation screw is advanced under fluoroscopy, and lead measurements are taken in a similar fashion. Generally acceptable parameters include P waves over 2.0 millivolts and a threshold under two volts at 0.4 ms with a stable impedance. Similar to ventricular lead placement, a large current of injury is desirable. In patients with significant right atrial dilation and scarring, other locations such as the lateral wall or septum may be required due to poor parameters at initial sites. Once an adequate sight is obtained, slack is also placed in this lead, and the suture sleeve is tied down to the pectoralis muscle in a similar fashion.

After lead placement, the pocket is vigorously irrigated with saline and hemostasis in the pocket is confirmed. The leads are then connected to the device. The excess leads are coiled around the device and then both are placed into the pocket, making sure to avoid sharp turns, which can place excess stress on the leads. The device is usually secured to the pectoralis muscle with silk suture in order to prevent device migration. The pocket is then closed with absorbable suture and layers. Either surgical adhesive or Steri-Strips are applied to the incision.

Several hours after the procedure, a chest X-ray is performed to exclude the presence of pneumothorax as well as to examine placement of the leads. Interrogation is also performed to be sure pacing parameters and function are acceptable. Patients are advised to avoid excessive movements of the upper extremity for approximately 4 weeks to avoid lead dislodgement. Patients are often discharged the same day if the procedure is performed in the outpatient setting. Outpatient follow-up is usually done in approximately 1 month to assess the implant site as well as to perform device interrogation and set chronic pacing parameters.

Implantable Cardio Defibrillator (ICD) Guidelines

Reasons for implanting an ICD can be broken down into primary and secondary prevention of sudden cardiac arrest. While initial implants were done for patients who had survived cardiac arrest, most implants nowadays are in those patients who meet a primary prevention indication. These are patients who are at high risk for sudden cardiac arrest with the majority of patients being those have either ischemic or non-ischemic cardiomyopathy with LVEF below 35%. Other patients with conditions such as hypertrophic cardiomyopathy, infiltrative diseases or inherited arrhythmia syndromes may also qualify for ICD implants. A more comprehensive discussion of indications can be found in the 2017 AHA/ACC/HRS Guideline for Management of Patients with Ventricular Arrhythmias and the Prevention of Sudden Cardiac Death: Executive Summary.

ICD Implant

The technique to implant a transvenous ICD system is similar to that of pacemaker implantation as discussed above. As the device is bigger a larger incision and pocket is required. In patients who likely will not require much ventricular pacing, apical-septal placement is preferred. Mid septal sites can also be acceptable as long as enough of the ICD coil is in the right ventricle and atrial signals are not seen in systems with extended bipolar sensing configuration. Mid septal sites may be preferable for patients who require ventricular pacing and in patients where cardiac resynchronization therapy is also going to be performed. It is preferred that only single chamber ICD implants be performed if atrial pacing is not required.

Defibrillation Threshold Testing

The obvious goal of ICD implant is to terminate ventricular arrhythmias when required. Defibrillation threshold testing (DFT) is defined as the minimum energy required to successfully terminate ventricular arrythmia. Historically, DFT testing was performed to ensure a device would function appropriately in achieving this goal. The practice comes from the era of surgically placed epicardial patches and has been carried forward to modern day transvenous ICD implants. While risks of DFT remain quite low, more recent data and contemporary practice has gone away from defibrillation threshold testing as an absolute in patients with adequate sensing, impedance and pacing parameters and appropriate lead placement on fluoroscopy [4]. Many studies have not shown a long-term mortality benefit of doing DFT testing at the time of implant. Absolute contraindications include patients with intracardiac thrombus, severe aortic stenosis, hemodynamic instability, and atrial fibrillation/flutter patients off anticoagulation. In select cases it may be preferred to perform DFT testing such as right sided device implants or generator changes.

ICD Programming

Programming treatment parameters of the ICD should be focused on reducing the amount of inappropriate shocks while being able to deliver effective therapies for appropriate ventricular arrhythmias. It's important to realize that many ventricular arrhythmias may be non-sustained and not require ICD therapies and therefore prolonged detection times (>6 s) should be considered. The strategy significantly reduces inappropriate shocks as well as therapies for non-sustained arrhythmias while also providing the benefits of reduced morbidity and mortality. Programming also involves the selection of a rate cut-off for treatment. In patients who have an ICD implanted for primary prevention, we generally follow the "high rate" programming as done in the MADIT-RIT trial with a monitor zone beginning at 170 beats per minute and treatment zone starting at 200 beats per minute. In patients who have an ICD implanted for secondary prevention, we generally program treatment onset at approximately 10 beats below the known ventricular tachycardia cycle length [5].

SVT (atrial fibrillation/flutter, reentrant SVT, focal tachycardia) is a common cause of inappropriate shocks. Defibrillators have discriminator algorithms which can be programmed. These rely on several observations including ventricular beats greater than atrial beats, onset of arryhthmia, far field morphology discrimination, and regularity of tachycardia. However, if a tachycardia persists for a prolonged duration these discriminators may time out, and inappropriate shocks may result. Therefore, aggressive treatment of SVT with medications and preferably catheter ablation is recommended when it occurs in patients with ICDs.

Cardiac Resynchronization Therapy (CRT)

In patients with significant cardiomyopathy with left ventricular ejection fraction below 35% in the presence of conduction system disease, primarily left bundle branch block, there is dyssynchrony of ventricular contraction. Adding left ventricular pacing to a dual chamber pacemaker/ICD can help resynchronize ventricular contraction resulting in improvements in LV systolic function, improvement in mitral regurgitation, and acute hemodynamic benefits. Longer term improvements in left ventricular remodeling have also been noted. This coincides with improvements in heart failure and mortality outcomes as seen in landmark long term studies and trials such as COMPANION, MADIT-CRT, REVERSE, RAFT, and CARE-HF [6].

The decision to proceed with CRT centers on a wide QRS duration which ideally should be a left bundle branch block greater than 130 milliseconds along with a left ventricular ejection fraction below 35% and NYHA class II-IV symptoms. Patients should first be optimally treated with medical therapy at least greater than 3 months and reversible factors of cardiomyopathy should be excluded (ischemia, valvular disease, myocarditis etc.). CRT is also a consideration in patients who have LVEF between 35% and 50% who also have a pacing indication and are expected to pace greater than 40% of the time. Caution should be taken in recommending CRT in patients with non-left bundle branch block less than 150 ms as this patient population does not significantly benefit. It may be considered in these cases with patients who have refractory NYHA class III-IV heart failure and hospitalizations despite optimal medical therapy.

CRT Implantation Technique

The initial implant procedure proceeds in a similar fashion as described previously with an extra venous access obtained for left ventricular lead placement. Specialized coronary access sheaths have been developed which are placed over a long wire into the right ventricle. The sheath is gently withdrawn with counterclockwise torque which helps it point towards the coronary sinus ostium. Probing in this area with a glidewire will often lead to coronary sinus access and distal advancement of the wire (Fig. 4.2). Once stability is provided, the sheath can be advanced into the mid portion of the coronary sinus. If this is not initially successful a coronary sinus catheter can be used to map atrial and

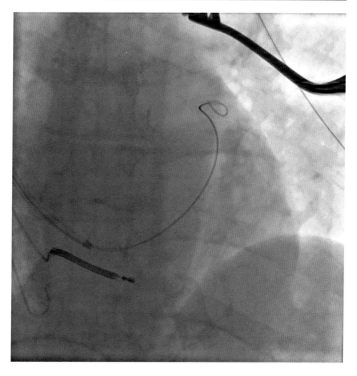

Fig. 4.2 Coronary sinus access with the glidewire in the main body of the CS and access sheath at the ostium prior to distal advancement

ventricular signals and once advanced into the CS help support distal sheath placement. Once the sheath is stable in the midportion of the CS, a coronary sinus balloon venogram is performed. This allows for identifications of suitable side branches for lead placement. It is preferred to place the lead in a lateral location which allows for sufficient separation from the right ventricular pacing lead (Fig. 4.3). Placement into the anterior interventricular vein as well as distal placement should be avoided as resynchronization will not be optimal. Once a suitable side branch is located a firm inner wire (Whisper wire) is used to sub-select the branch of interest and acts as a rail to advance the lead into the venous branch. Depending on the venous anatomy, different shapes and

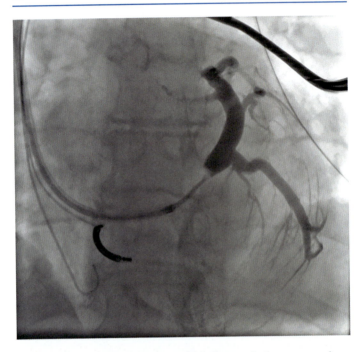

Fig. 4.3 Coronary Sinus Venogram with balloon occlusive venogram in an LAO view showing a large lateral side branch with distal bifurcation

styles of left ventricular leads are available for selection. Modern leads are quadrapolar, which allows for various pacing configurations to optimize pacing site, threshold, and battery usage (Fig. 4.4). The left phrenic nerve courses over the lateral portion of the left ventricle and testing for phrenic nerve stimulation should also be performed. It's possible that phrenic nerve stimulation is positional, and patients, later after the procedure is complete, may report phrenic nerve stimulation. Reprogramming of pacing configurations may be needed. Once the lead is in a satisfactory position, the inner wire is removed, and the coronary sinus access sheath is either peeled or cut away.

4 Implantable Cardiac Devices

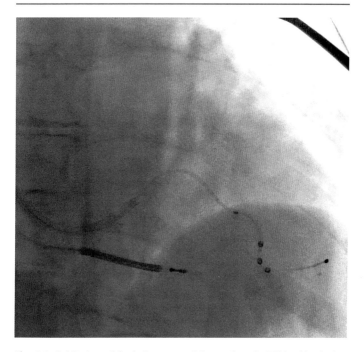

Fig. 4.4 RAO view of final placement of the quadrapolar LV lead in the lateral branch of interest

Subcutaneous Implantable Cardiac defibrillator (S-ICD)

Approved in 2012, the first subcutaneous ICD has offered an alternative to the traditional transvenous ICD which has been the standard [7]. The PRAETORIAN study evaluated 849 patients split in a nonrandomized 1:1 ratio between the S-ICD and transvenous ICD patients who had an indication for ICD therapy but did not have a pacing indication. The study showed that with respect to complications and inappropriate shocks the S-ICD was noninferior to the transvenous ICD.

The device is extra-thoracic with one coil implanted above the sternum and the ICD can in the midaxillary region. Given that it is extra-thoracic and extravascular it provides significant benefits for patients who do not have transvenous access. Additionally, given that it is outside the vascular system and not subject to the stresses of a lifetime of cardiac contraction, lead infection/endocarditis risk as well as lead fracture become less of an issue. When compared to traditional transvenous ICD leads, in the ATLAS trial, the Boston Scientific EMBLEM™ S-ICD system showed a 92% reduction in serious lead related complications at 6 months.

In the UNTOUCHED trial (Understanding Outcomes With the S-ICD in Primary Prevention Patients With Low Ejection Fraction) over 1100 patients were followed for 18 months. Most notable was the low rate of inappropriate shocks (3.1% at 1 year) using contemporary programming with success rates for appropriate therapy delivery at 98.4%.

In the subsequent generation, the S-ICD has become smaller, and battery technology has provided more longevity. It is particularly an attractive option for patients who do not have a pacing need, or younger and have infection risk. However, given that it is not intracardiac, Defibrillation requires higher energy, and patients must pass screening to be sure that QRS sensing is adequate so that effective therapy can be sensed and delivered. Additionally, anti-tachycardia pacing cannot be delivered by the device, although pairing with a leadless pacemaker may potentially become an option in the future.

The ICD can is placed in the midaxillary region of the left chest ideally in an intramuscular location between the latissimus dorsi and the serratus anterior (Fig. 4.5). Placement in this intramuscular location improves cosmesis and may help lower Defibrillation threshold. It is important to be sure that the can is placed posterior enough so that the shocking vector covers the cardiac profile. Initial superficial placement as viewed on fluoroscopy can be helpful. The lead is tunneled on anterior to the sternum from a near subxiphoid location towards the sternal notch. From the lower chest the lead is then tunneled towards the midaxillary region and connected to the device. The system then provides multiples vectors for QRS sensing.

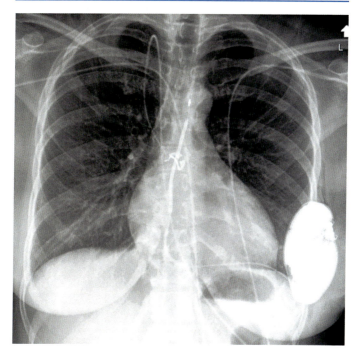

Fig. 4.5 PA CXR view of the S-ICD system with the can located in the mid axillary region and the shocking coil on the sternum. Sensing for arrhythmia detection can be done 3 ways

Leadless Pacemaker

While millions of people worldwide have benefitted from implantation of transvenous pacemaker systems, the traditional system consisting of a generator and lead has weaknesses [8]. The lead is subject to the constant repetitive stress of cardiac contraction as well as possible stress of upper body movements. Over time, this can lead to insulation breach and lead fracture. The right ventricular lead crosses the tricuspid valve and although rare, can result in severe tricuspid valve regurgitation. The generator, implanted in the upper chest, on occasion may erode through the chest, particularly in patients with a lack of subcutaneous tissue. Additionally, this foreign object within the body can serve as a harbor for systemic infections, requiring a risky extraction procedure. Lastly, the traditional pacemaker system requires venous access which may at times be compromised in certain patients.

The recent advent of a leadless pacemaker has potential to address these issues. With the entire small unit (Medtronic Micra 0.8^{cm3}/Abbott Aveir VR 1.0^{cm3}) implanted in the right ventricle containing the generator as well as pacing mechanism, no separate incision has to be made in the upper chest, and the venous system does not contain a lead [9]. Additionally, the tricuspid valve is not compromised, as the entire system is implanted in the right ventricle. Early data also shows infection rates of leadless pacemakers occur at several magnitudes lower than traditional transvenous systems.

Concerns of the leadless pacemaker include learning a separate implant procedure, removal of the system in rare cases when it is needed, and the need to add another device when the first one is at the end of its life. Additionally, as the device is implanted into right ventricle only right ventricular pacing is possible. The Medtronic Micra AV device can sense atrial contraction and pace the ventricle in a synchronous fashion. Currently in clinical trials, implantation of a device in the atrium as well as one in the ventricle will allow for DDD pacing. Also, pairing a leadless device with a subcutaneous ICD is a potentially evolving technology which will allow for intracardiac sensing and the delivery of anti-tachycardia pacing for the treatment of ventricular arrhythmia.

Currently, two leadless devices are commercially available, the Medtronic Micra system and the Abbott Aveir VR system (Figs. 6 and 7). Both devices are implanted in a similar fashion. A large sheath in the femoral vein is advanced into the right heart. Through this, the device which is mounted on a delivery platform is advanced into the right ventricle through the sheath (Fig. 4.6a). Once a suitable location is found (Fig. 4.6b), the device is deployed and tested. We prefer a more septal placement to reduce the risk of free wall or apical perforation. The Medtronic system has four distal nitinol tines which grab into the trabeculated myocardium to secure its fixation while the Abbott Aveir VR system

4 Implantable Cardiac Devices

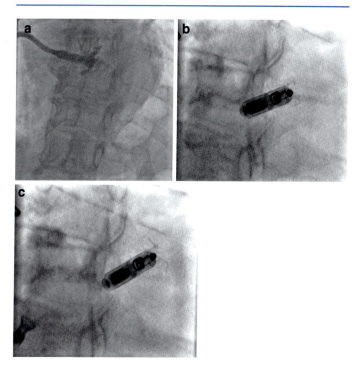

Fig. 4.6 (**a, b, c**) Delivery and zoomed view of a final position of a Medtronic Micra leadless pacemaker. In Figure (**a**) a contrast injection is performed to ensure a septal position to aid in delivery and device fixation. In Figures (**b**) and (**c**) 2 out of 4 tines are clearly visible in these views. (**b**) shows the fixation without tension and 8c when the tether (not visible under fluoroscopy) is pulled. Note the flexing of the tines in (**c**). At least 2 out of the 4 tines should flex when the tether is gently pulled to ensure adequate fixation prior to the tether being cut and released. Multiple views with fluoroscopy may be necessary to visualize the different tines

has a screw-in helix. Once fixation and testing is satisfactory a tether is cut and the delivery system is removed. Both devices have a proximal anchor which allows for a retrieval system or snare to attach to and retrieve the device when rarely necessary.

Complications of the device procedure are mainly related to cardiac perforation and subsequent tamponade. Venous injury is also a possibility given the large sheath. Device dislodgement is a very rare possibility as well. Complications of perforation trended lower as operator experience improved. Long term complications when compared to the traditional transvenous system was also lower by several fold in observational studies and comparison to historical cohorts as there is no generator or transvenous lead.

Conduction System Pacing

To review briefly, in a normal heart, depolarization of the ventricle occurs when an impulse from the sinus node is received by the AV node. The impulse then travels through the bundle of His, followed by the left and right bundle branches. The bundle branches depolarize their respective ventricles via the Purkinje system. Individual myocytes are also capable of spreading action potentials but do so more slowly than the bundle branches. When bundle branch block is present, the corresponding ventricle will depolarize slowly via myocyte conduction. In traditional RV pacing, left bundle branch block physiology is created: the myocytes of the heart are being activated by the pacing stimulus from the lead placed in the apical septum.

As previously outlined, traditional ventricular pacing involves placement of a lead in the mid- to distal right ventricular septum. While this results in capture of myocardial tissue, resulting electrical propagation through slow-conducting myocardium is not physiologic and ventricular function is dyssynchronous and may lead to LV dysfunction [10]. While biventricular pacing helps with resynchronization by depolarizes the LV myocardium by way of a lead in the coronary sinus, pacing in this manner is still not physiologic as the native His-Purkinje system is still not utilized. In some patients with a high burden of ventricular pacing, detrimental effects of long-term right ventricular (RV) pacing can lead to left ventricular (LV) systolic dysfunction known as pacemaker mediated cardiomyopathy. The DAVID trial showed a significant increase in mortality with dual-chamber ICD placement, suggesting that an increased burden of RV pacing in DDD devices may increase incidence of heart failure exacerbation [11]. Over time electrophysiologists have sought other methods for pacing that can utilize natural conduction and preserve ventricular synchrony [12]. This method of conduction system pacing involves placing a lead that primarily pacing the bundle of His or the left bundle branch resulting in myocardial stimulation by more physiologic means.

His-Bundle Pacing

In 2000, Deshmukh and colleagues demonstrated the feasibility of placing a His-bundle lead in a small group of patients with chronic atrial fibrillation, cardiomyopathy, and heart failure [13]. After lead insertion, most patients had a QRS interval that was close to baseline, reflecting successful His bundle capture. Some patients underwent AVJ ablation for fast ventricular rates. A statistically significant increase in LVEF was observed, perhaps reflecting improved synchrony as a cause; however, results may have been confounded by better rate-control. Nevertheless, the feasibility of the strategy was established, prompting further study in the field [13]. In 2017, Sharma et al. demonstrated that His bundle pacing was a viable rescue strategy for patients in whom a coronary sinus lead for biventricular pacing could not be successfully placed. Placing the His-bundle lead still led to a statistically significant improvement in LVEF and New York Heart Association heart failure class [14]. Subsequently, in 2018, Arnold and colleagues demonstrated that His bundle pacing yields a narrower QRS, better ventricular synchrony, and a better hemodynamic profile than biventricular pacing during EP studies on a small cohort of patients [15].

Implanting a His-bundle lead involves first obtaining standard access through the axillary or subclavian vein, using a J-tip wire. Over the wire, a specialized sheath is advanced to the tricuspid annulus. The sheath has a curve designed to direct toward the RV septum. Once the sheath is positioned properly, the pacing lead is inserted through the sheath. The sheath and wire are then manipulated until a His-bundle potential is identified. Then the lead is gently screwed into the myocardium.

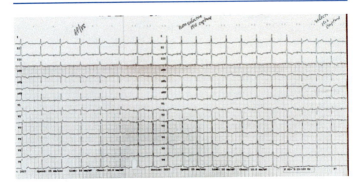

Fig. 4.7 Continuous 12-lead rhythm strip showing intrinsic QRS complex (AP/VS), non-selective His capture and selective His capture during threshold testing. With non-selective His capture there is a slight "delta" complex after the pacing spike reflecting some

Thresholds for pacing are tested; a threshold of <2.0 mV at a pulse width of 1 ms is generally desired. Capture may be selective (only the His bundle is captured) or non-selective (the His bundle and adjacent myocardium are both captured (Fig. 4.7)); both selective and non-selective capture have similar hemodynamic benefits [12]. Selective and nonselective capture are distinguished by QRS duration; in selective capture, a short isoelectric interval is present after the pacing stimulus and the QRS is more narrow, similar to the patient's baseline (Fig. 4.7) A slighter wider QRS is seen with nonselective capture due to surrounding myocardial capture which fuses with His capture and native conduction system propagation.

Despite its promise for improving ventricular synchrony, His bundle pacing has several limitations. First, the premise for successful capture relies upon the patient having more proximal disease. If more distal conduction disease is present, successful QRS narrowing is less likely to be achieved although in many cases a sufficient output can overcome local conduction block [12]. The His bundle location is also extremely narrow, and thus is a small window for adequate capture [16]. As a result, His bundle leads often have higher thresholds, which can lead to decreased battery life [17].

Left Bundle Branch Pacing

Considering the technical challenges seen with His-bundle pacing, as outlined above, alternative targets for conduction system pacing were sought. The proximal left bundle and deep septum offer more forgiving targets for lead placement, as well as lower thresholds. There is also a "backup" built in as surrounding myocardium can still be captured in case the conduction system is not. Additionally, animal studies demonstrated favorable hemodynamic profiles with left bundle and septal pacing, when compared with RV-only pacing [18]. The distinction between left bundle pacing and deep septal pacing lies in which tissue is captured. In deep septal pacing, predominantly myocardium is captured; in true left bundle branch pacing, the proximal left bundle fibers are captured, in addition to adjacent myocardium [18]. Left bundle branch area pacing, as well as deep septal pacing, also typically has lower thresholds (<1.0 mV at a pulse width of 0.4 ms) than His bundle pacing, preserving device battery life [19].

The lead and sheath most used for left bundle pacing are the same as those for His-bundle pacing (Medtronic 3830 lead, with a C315 His sheath) although other companies have started introducing selective pacing tools as well. Huang et al. described the technique for successful left bundle capture in a 2019 issue of Heart Rhythm [20]. The His position is initially identified, after transvenous access is obtained (typically via an axillary/subclavian route, as with His bundle pacing.) Then, the sheath is advanced to a position about 1–1.5 cm distal to the His position on the LV septum. The lead is then burrowed into the septum using counterclockwise rotation. The QRS morphology is then examined in a unipolar configuration. Ideally, the QRS complex should have a qR morphology in lead V1, and a peak left ventricular activation time (the time from the pacing spike to the peak of the R-wave) of less than 80 ms in leads V5 and V6, which is consistent with quick lateral LV activation [17].

Complications of left bundle branch pacing include septal perforation into the LV, damage to the right bundle, and injury to septal perforator arteries [16]. To prevent placing the lead too far into the septum, the impedance on the lead is watched closely during placement, as well as the QRS morphology. The impedance should not drop below 500 Ohms; if it does, the suspicion for perforation is raised [20].

Until recently, no head-to-head comparisons have been made between left bundle selective pacing and traditional CRT with a coronary sinus lead. However, in an August 2022 edition of Heart Rhythm, Vijayaraman and colleagues at Geisinger Health and Rush University published an observational study examining outcomes of patients who had undergone CRT and conduction system pacing at their centers. The patients who underwent conduction system pacing, as compared to CRT, had lower rates of a combined primary endpoint: heart failure hospitalizations and mortality. With conduction system pacing, a statistically significant greater reduction in QRS duration was observed, as well as a greater increase in left ventricular ejection fraction. Although randomized controlled trials are needed to make more definitive conclusions, these initial findings are encouraging [21]. As it stands currently, we strongly prefer conduction system pacing in patients who are expected to have a high burden of ventricular pacing and in those CRT patients in whom attempts at LV pacing are unsuccessful.

Device Interrogation

Device implantation is the first step for a patient who needs device therapy. Over time, the device needs to be interrogated on a routine basis or at times where there are concerns for symptoms or device malfunction [22].

An interrogation is the ability of a **CIED** (cardiac implantable electronic device) to communicate wirelessly with a programmer by placing a "wand" over the device site. The information is gathered from the device's memory and displayed for viewing. This session also allows for programming of the device when done in person. Most patients now have remote interrogation capabilities where "read only" information can be gathered from the device from a transmitter at home. Remote programming cannot be performed. However, this is an attractive feature for the patient care team to have timely access to routine information as well as be alerted for any device malfunctions or significant arrhythmias without having to see the patient in person.

4 Implantable Cardiac Devices

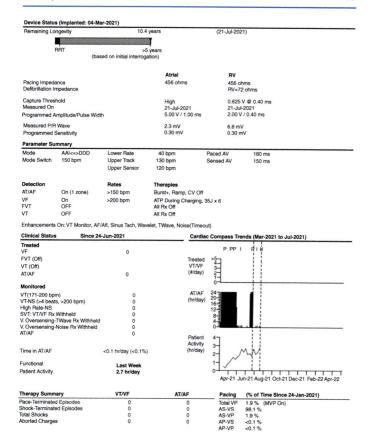

Fig. 4.8 Interrogation summary page (Medtronic)

An interrogation report contains a wealth of information. Patient data, including name and date of birth, implanting physician, and place of implant are recorded under patient information tab. Special notes can be written here as well to convey any pertinent information.

Although formatting is different for various manufacturers, the main page (Fig. 4.8) generally shows alerts, battery status, diagnostics, settings and lead measurements (thresholds, impedance and sensing.)

Device Interrogation Session

Our usual complete device interrogation (Fig. 4.9) process involves the following.

1. Review alerts which can point out any concerns with device function and any concerning arrhythmias.
2. View the presenting and underlying rhythm.
3. Check battery status for longevity estimates. Total battery life is estimated anywhere from 8–15 years depending on usage. The elective replacement indicator (**ERI**) means there are approximately 3 months of battery life left.
4. Assess lead performance including manual examination for sensing, threshold and impedance values and review the recorded trends over time.

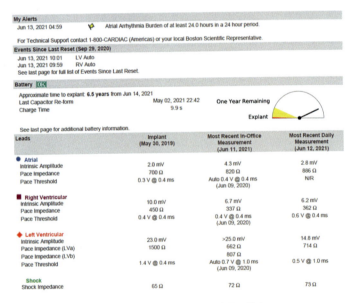

Fig. 4.9 Interrogation summary page (Boston Scientific)

5. Review the arrhythmia logbook and saved electrograms. This can be helpful in managing patients who have burden of arrhythmia such as atrial fibrillation or ventricular tachycardia.
6. Examination of heart rate histograms, percentage of pacing, rate response performance, PVC burden and percentage of left ventricular pacing (for CRT devices)
7. Heart failure sensors (in applicable devices)
8. Examination of the device site, especially with recent implant or symptoms.

Assessing lead performance involves looking at the sensing, threshold, and impendence. Pacemakers can be programmed to pace and sense in a bipolar or unipolar mode. Intrinsic conduction is tested by decreasing the patient's rate below the rate at which they are currently pacing assuming they are not pacemaker dependent.

Sensing intrinsic conduction is one main function of a pacemaker or ICD, as it will inhibit pacing and allow tachyarrhythmia therapy to be delivered in the case of an ICD. In cases where sensing is not appropriate, identification and remedy is essential to avoid device malfunction. The causative issue could be related to an external factor or with the device itself. Programming sensitivity in the device is usually less than half of the measured P wave or R wave in a pacemaker and a nominal setting in an ICD so that ventricular fibrillatory waves are sensed when needed.

Sensing extraneous electrical activity from anything other than electrical signal of interest is referred to as oversensing and can lead to problems of pacing inhibition in a pacemaker and inappropriate delivery of anti-tachycardia pacing or ICD shock in an ICD. Examples include EMI (electro-magnetic interference), T wave oversensing (Fig. 4.10) or myopotentials (Fig. 4.11), or lead fracture (Fig. 4.12).

The opposite can also be a problem which is called undersensing (Fig. 4.13). With this, the device does not appropriately sense an intrinsic beat and can lead to overpacing in a pacemaker and failure to deliver therapy in an ICD. Some examples related to undersensing include lead dislodgement, electrolyte abnormalities, local infarction, and cardiomyopathy.

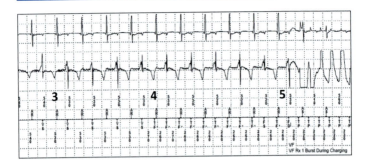

Fig. 4.10 T wave over sensing (TF) causing inappropriate ICD therapies as device believes it to be VT

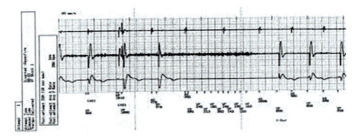

Fig. 4.11 Oversensing myopotentials causing inhibition of pacing, labelled as VF

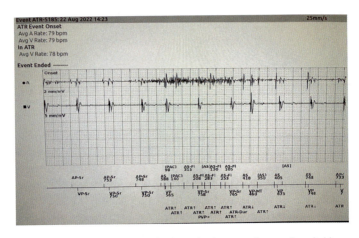

Fig. 4.12 Lead fracture on RA lead causing inappropriate mode switching

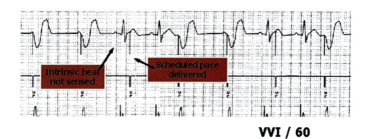

Fig. 4.13 Undersensing in a pacemaker leading to pacer spikes at inappropriate times

Examination of the intracardiac electrograms allows the provider to see what the device interprets and aids in making a diagnosis and remediating the issue. Some examples are below.

Threshold testing tests the least amount of energy it takes to pace that portion of the heart muscle to which the lead is in contact. This is referred to as capture. Lower voltage to capture helps preserve battery longevity. Outputs are the way the leads are programmed. They are measured in amplitude (voltage) and pulse width (milliseconds). Each lead has its own output programming. Once the threshold is tested, the voltage output should be doubled, or the milliseconds tripled at a set voltage to provide an adequate safety margin.

Most modern devices perform beat to beat autocapture, as the device is capable of sensing the evoked potential of myocardial capture. This feature allows a lower programming output to help save battery life while ensuring adequate pacing.

An increase in voltage requirements or loss of capture (Fig. 4.14) can be seen in lead fracture or dislodgement, electrolyte abnormalities, lead tip fibrosis, or anti-arrhythmic drugs (Na^+ channel blockers).

Pacing Lead impedance testing reflects the resistance of electrical flow through the lead. A usual range is 200-2000 ohms and specific for each lead type. If <200 ohms this can signify insulation breakdown. If >2000 ohms, then lead fracture is suspected when acute and development of fibrosis if the impedence chronically increases.

As shown in Fig. 4.15, reviewing heart rate trends and the arrhythmia logbook can give an insight into the patient's cardiac

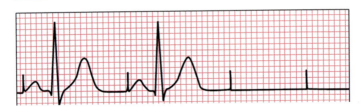

Fig. 4.14 A rhythm strip showing intermittent failure to capture in the atrium as seen by no P wave after a pacing spike

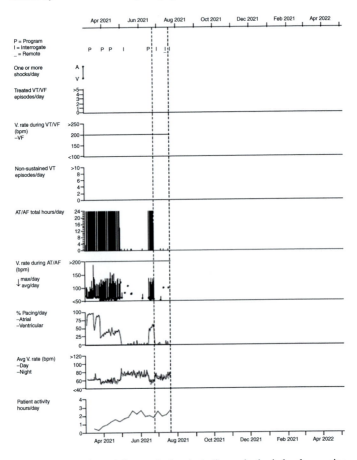

Fig. 4.15 Overview of diagnostic data including arrhythmia burden, pacing percentage and patient status

4 Implantable Cardiac Devices

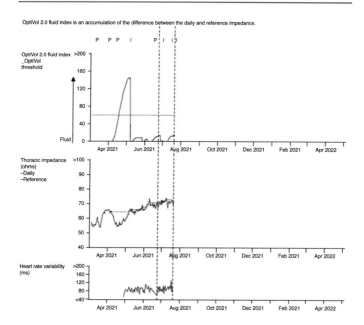

Fig. 4.16 In OptiVol, as the intrathoracic fluid increases, thoracic impedance decreases

profile. Much data can be gleaned which can help titrate medications and guide appropriate therapy recommendations.

Heart failure diagnostic information can be assessed on certain defibrillators, since fluid is a good conductor of electrical current. OptiVol fluid index, in Medtronic devices, measures intrathoracic impedance (Fig. 4.16). The impedance decreases as the amount of fluid in the lungs increases. Heart Logic Index (Fig. 4.17), in Boston Scientific devices utilizes 5 sensors—heart sounds, thoracic impedance, respiration, heart rate and activity. Abbott CorVue also measures intrathoracic impedance. These algorithms are meant to be used in concert with a clinical assessment as tools to help address heart failure status and impending heart failure episodes.

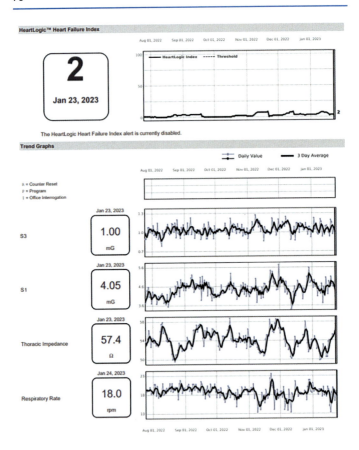

Fig. 4.17 Heart Logic (Boston Scientific) notes 5 sensors (not all shown in figure) and reports as an index. 16 and below is consistent with appropriate volume status

Devices record arrhythmias, such as SVT, AT, VT, AFib, or atrial flutter. These include a rhythm strip, time and date of the event, duration, average ventricular response/heart rate. Examination of the intracardiac electrograms can help with diagnosis and aid in tailoring therapy (Figs. 4.18, 4.19, 4.20).

4 Implantable Cardiac Devices

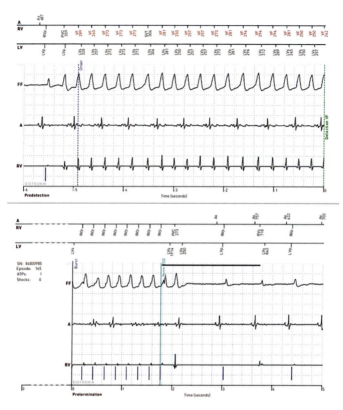

Fig. 4.18 Sustained VT, with successful ATP therapy avoiding the need for ICD shock

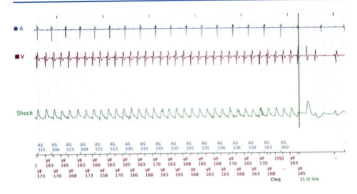

Fig. 4.19 Sustained rapid VT, resulting in ICD shock. Note more ventricular than atrial signals consistent with VT

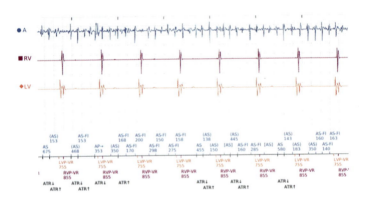

Fig. 4.20 Atrial fibrillation with demand ventricular pacing

Conclusion

Device based therapy has a primary role in the field of electrophysiology. From the extensive monitoring provided by an implantable cardiac monitor to the lifesaving capabilities of an implantable cardiac defibrillator these devices have helped millions of patients worldwide. Having a fundamental knowledge of the technology available will allow the treating provider to maximize the offerings currently available and take advantage of future innovations in this exciting field.

References

1. Kusumoto F, et al. 2018 ACC/AHA/HRS guideline on the evaluation and management of patients with bradycardia and cardiac conduction delay. Circulation. 2019;140:e382–482.
2. Goldberger Z, et al. ACC/AHA/HRS versus ESC guidelines for the diagnosis and management of syncope. J Am Coll Cardiol. 2019;74:2410–23.
3. Bisagnani A, et al. Implantable loop recorder in clinical practice. J Arrhythm. 2019;35:25–32.
4. Hayase J, et al. Defibrillation testing during ICD implantation—should we or should we not? JAFIB. 2017;9:5.
5. Wilkoff B, et al. 2015 HRS/EHRA/APHRS/SOLAECE expert consensus statement on optimal implantable cardioverter-defibrillator programming and testing. Europace. 2016;18:159–83.
6. Moss AJ, et al. Cardiac-resynchronization therapy for the prevention of heart-failure events. N Engl J Med. 2009;361(14):1329–38.
7. Kaya E, et al. Subcutaneous ICD: current standards and future perspective. IJC Heart Vasc. 2019;24:100409.
8. Madhavan M, et al. Advances and future directions in cardiac pacemakers. J Am Coll Cardiol. 2017;69:211–35.
9. Bencardino G, et al. Leadless pacemaker technology: clinical evidence of new paradigm of pacing. Rev Cardiovasc Med. 2022;23(2):043.
10. Naqvi TZ, Chao CJ. Adverse effects of right ventricular pacing on cardiac function: prevalence, prevention and treatment with physiologic pacing. Trends Cardiovasc Med. 2021;
11. Wilkoff BL, et al. Dual-chamber pacing or ventricular backup pacing in patients with an implantable defibrillator: the dual chamber and VVI implantable defibrillator (DAVID) trial. JAMA. 2002;288(24):3115–23.
12. Vijayaraman P, et al. His bundle pacing. J Am Coll Cardiol. 2018;72(8):927–47.
13. Deshmukh P, et al. Permanent, direct His-bundle pacing: a novel approach to cardiac pacing in patients with normal His-Purkinje activation. Circulation. 2000;101(8):869–77.
14. Sharma PS, et al. Permanent his-bundle pacing as an alternative to biventricular pacing for cardiac resynchronization therapy: a multicenter experience. Heart Rhythm. 2018;15(3):413–20.
15. Arnold AD, et al. His resynchronization versus biventricular pacing in patients with heart failure and left bundle branch block. J Am Coll Cardiol. 2018;72(24):3112–22.
16. Zhang S, Zhou X, Gold MR. Left bundle branch pacing: JACC review topic of the week. J Am Coll Cardiol. 2019;74(24):3039–49.
17. Ponnusamy SS, et al. Left bundle branch pacing: a comprehensive review. J Cardiovasc Electrophysiol. 2020;31(9):2462–73.
18. Wu S, Sharma PS, Huang W. Novel left ventricular cardiac synchronization: left ventricular septal pacing or left bundle branch pacing? Europace. 2020;22(Suppl_2):ii10–8.

19. Arnold AD, Whinnett ZI, Vijayaraman P. His-Purkinje conduction system pacing: state of the art in 2020. Arrhythm Electrophysiol Rev. 2020;9(3):136–45.
20. Huang W, et al. A beginner's guide to permanent left bundle branch pacing. Heart Rhythm. 2019;16(12):1791–6.
21. Vijayaraman P, et al. Clinical outcomes of conduction system pacing compared to biventricular pacing in patients requiring cardiac resynchronization therapy. Heart Rhythm. 2022;19(8):1263–71.
22. Mulpuru S, et al. Cardiac pacemakers: function, troubleshooting and management, part 1 of 2. J Am Coll Cardiol. 2017;69:189–210.

Diagnosis and Treatment of Supraventricular Tachycardias

Spencer Rosero and Travis Prinzi

Abstract

Supraventricular tachycardias are a group of arrhythmias that include atrio-ventricular nodal tachycardias (AVNRT), atrial tachycardia, and atrio-ventricular reentry tachycardias (AVRT) including Wolff-Parkinson-White Syndrome. Each of these arrhythmias, while originating in the upper chambers of the heart, involve various diagnostic maneuvers to determine their exact origin and treatment. Some will require simple pacing maneuvers to determine diagnosis, while others will involve complex, high density mapping from advanced mapping systems and algorithms in order to precisely treat the arrhythmia's origin. Careful attention must be given to differential diagnostic maneuvers and to 3D map interpretation.

Keywords

Supraventricular tachycardia · Atrial tachycardia · Atrioventricular nodal reentrant tachycardia · Atrio-ventricular tachycardia · Accessory pathways · Atrial tachycardia · Ablation 3D mapping · Pacing maneuvers

---

S. Rosero (✉) · T. Prinzi
University of Rochester Medical Center, Rochester, NY, USA
e-mail: Spencer_Rosero@urmc.Rochester.edu

© The Author(s), under exclusive license to Springer Nature Switzerland AG 2023
D. T. Huang et al. (eds.), *Cardiac Electrophysiology in Clinical Practice*, In Clinical Practice,
https://doi.org/10.1007/978-3-031-41479-4_5

The purpose of this chapter is to provide a basic overview of the mechanisms, management and practical considerations in the electrophysiology laboratory.

Introduction

Supraventricular tachycardias are a group of arrhythmias that include atrio-ventricular nodal tachycardias (AVNRT), atrial tachycardia, and atrio-ventricular reentry tachycardias (AVRT) including Wolff-Parkinson-White Syndrome. The purpose of this chapter is to provide a basic overview of the mechanisms, management and practical considerations in the electrophysiology laboratory.

Atrioventricular Nodal Reentry

The most common type of SVT is atrioventricular nodal reentry (AVNRT), accounting for the majority of diagnosed SVT in patients under 50 years, with a higher prevalence in women compared to men. Quality of life has also been shown to be affected in various populations [1, 2]. Clinical ECG demonstrates a short RP, narrow complex tachycardia with evidence of retrograde conduction seen as a pseudo S wave with a superior axis P waves (Fig. 5.1).

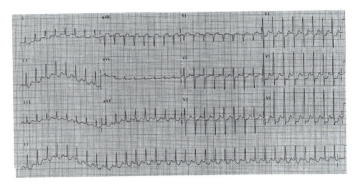

Fig. 5.1 ECG of AVNRT. Notice retrograde P waves forming a pseudo S pattern in several leads

5 Diagnosis and Treatment of Supraventricular Tachycardias

This short RP tachycardia involves a reentry mechanism within the AV node and is based on the concept of dual AV nodal physiology . The reentrant circuit is dependent on the presence of at least two functional pathways with differing refractoriness and conduction properties. Typical AVNRT, the most frequent form, uses the slow pathway for antegrade conduction, and the fast pathway for retrograde limb to complete the circuit and is classically triggered by an APC blocking in the fast pathway but conducting slowly down the slow pathway allowing retrograde recovery of the fast pathway to produce a closed loop (Fig. 5.2) [3, 4].

The two pathways do not seem separable by pathologic examination but the characteristics are encoded within the cellular distribution, and the characteristics for electrophysiology properties are functional [4–6]. The differentiation of function within the AV node was originally discovered from analyzing atrial pacing data using progressively shorter atrial extrastimuli cycle lengths (A1-A2) and measuring the A-H conduction times, during which it was noted that a large "jump" of at least 50 msec occurred at a specific 10 ms decrement in A1-A2 cycle length after which the resumption of gradual normal decremental conduction would continue on a different slope (Fig. 5.3). This reproducible finding confirmed the functional presence of dual pathway physiology

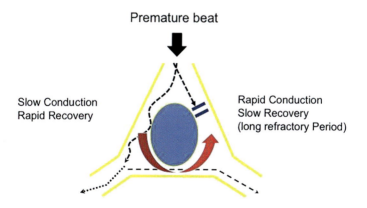

Fig. 5.2 Diagram of dual pathway physiology within the AV node and initiation via an APC

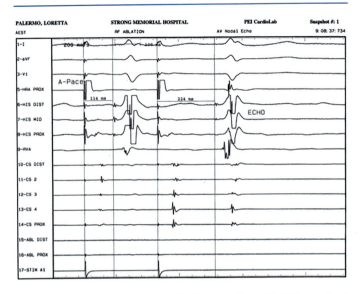

Fig. 5.3 Paced atrial extrastimuli with subsequent "jump" in AH interval and one beat reentry. This is referred to as an echo

and provides the substrate for a reentry based tachycardia such as AVNRT. This mechanism also explains the surface ECG findings of an APC with sudden PR prolongation preceding initiation of a short RP tachycardia with evidence of retrograde P wave conduction. The intracardiac findings confirm a jump in AH interval meeting the dual pathway criteria with initiation of a short RP tachycardia.

The atrial electrogram on the His catheter is earliest since the return limb in the typical form involves the anterior pathway located close to the anteroseptal region.

The fast and slow pathways are considered to anatomically located within the triangle of Koch during which the earliest retrograde conduction to the atrium is noted. In typical AVNRT, the earliest retrograde atrial activation EGM is noted in the apex of the triangle, and in the OS of the coronary sinus during the atypical form. It is important to note that not all cases of AVNRT demonstrate clear dual AV nodal physiology during baseline EP studies, since the "jump" is heavily influenced by timing and autonomic tone.

Clinical Presentation

Patients with AVNRT often present with a history of paroxysmal palpitations, that may be triggered after bending down to pickup a heavy object, or preceded by a sensation of single "skipped beats". It is interesting to note that many adolescent patients instinctively perform their own vagal maneuvers to terminate the SVT including bearing down or less commonly, standing on their head terminating the tachycardia via vagal like mechanism. Adults may describe a history of palpitations during their teenage years, the frequency of which may have decreased for many years, only to return later in life. While the tachycardia cycle length may decrease in a subgroup of patients with age, the ability to tolerate the fast rates may not. Common symptoms include sudden onset and termination, sensation of racing or palpitations, chest heaviness or unusual sensation in neck and throat prompting a cough. While the SVT may last only minutes, it may be prolonged and incessant prompting an emergency room visit. Intravenous adenosine is often used in the pre-hospital and hospital setting with excellent success in terminating the tachycardia.

Clinical Management

There are three decision pathways: Observation, Pharmacologic, and Catheter ablation. The individual patient's circumstances need to be included in the process. For example, a single episode of SVT and no history of symptoms may benefit from observation or event monitoring with no pharmacologic or invasive intervention. Catheter ablation is generally curative and is the preferred path for patients with recurrent episodes that are symptomatic, limited by possibility of having prolonged episodes requiring emergency services, and/or occupation that may increase patient risk for injury should he or she develop sustained SVT that is symptomatic. Pharmacologic management primarily rely on drugs such as beta receptor and calcium channel antagonists that modulate AV node function to reduce the probability of SVT events over long periods of time. The next level of pharmacologic intervention would include antiarrhythmics such as flecainide or propafenone, which concomitantly have a higher side effect profile.

Electrophysiology Study and Ablation

Several forms of AVNRT have been described during EP studies including slow-fast (typical) and fast-slow (atypical). The correct diagnosis is critical to determining if and where an RF ablation should be delivered. The goal is to eliminate the appropriate limb of the reentry circuit while minimizing risk to the normal conduction system. When performing the EP study for SVT, it is important to maintain a systematic approach to avoid missing key maneuvers and improving your diagnostic accuracy. We recommend that physicians customize and adopt a framework on which to approach all EP studies. The following is only an example of possible considerations during an EP study:

1. Document baseline sinus rhythm, AH, HV intervals. Any pre-excitation? Is the AV conduction normal?
2. 1:1 A-V conduction
3. AV node function –Effective refractory periods using programmed stimulation
4. Any evidence of dual AV nodal physiology? (Fig. 5.3)
5. 1:1 V-A conduction: Is it concentric? Is it decremental?
6. Parahisian pacing (Fig. 5.4)
7. Attempt burst pacing and varying atrial and ventricular extrastimuli.
8. Add agents such as isoproterenol or atropine to alter autonomic tone to increase the probability of inducing SVT.

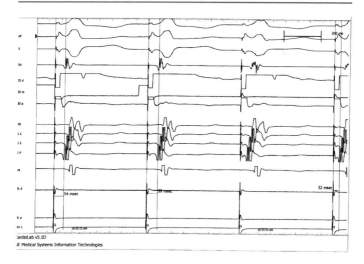

Fig. 5.4 Example of ParaHisian pacing

In typical AVNRT, the ECG reveals a short RP narrow complex regular tachycardia in which the P wave is buried within the terminal segment of the QRS complex and not clearly visible. Intracardiac electrograms demonstrate that the earliest retrograde activation is often seen on the His Bundle electrode, though it may be occasionally seen earlier along the posterior septum (Fig. 5.5)). The QA interval is relatively short. One must always consider the less probable presence of a left sided fast pathway.

Pacing maneuvers during tachycardia are powerful tools for correctly diagnosing the circuit. For example, rapid ventricular pacing causing dissociation between the atrium and ventricle provides a clue. In this setting, the atrial cycle length remains unchanged thus ruling out AVRT as the etiology of the ongoing tachycardia but does not rule out arrhythmias such as atrial tachycardia. Another maneuver during 1:1 conduction involves introducing single premature ventricular beats at a time during His refractoriness and determining if it resets the atrial activation. Parahisian pacing also aids in determining the presence of a concealed septal bypass tract [7, 8].

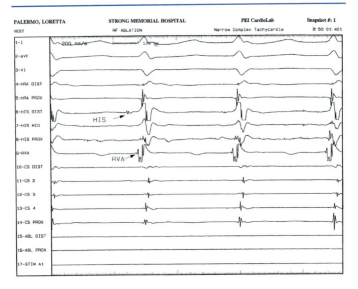

Fig. 5.5 Atrioventricular nodal reentry tachycardia

It is important to recognize that there is a small but real risk of damaging the AV node fast pathway causing high grade AV block that may be irreversible. Fluoroscopic views maximizing the distance between the anteroseptum and the posteroseptal region near the coronary sinus where the slow pathway is localized reduces risk. Additionally, 3D mapping in which the His bundle is carefully marked can reduce risk. During RF delivery, monitoring VA conduction during junctional beats as well as the A-H-V conduction during sinus will provide clues to unintended conduction system damage.

Atrial Tachycardia

Atrial tachycardias originate from cells depolarizing within the atria and function independently of the AV node conduction system and ventricle. The anatomic site of origin can be anywhere in the left and right atria. An atrial tachycardia may originate from

5 Diagnosis and Treatment of Supraventricular Tachycardias

one or more foci and presents on ECG as an SVT with evidence of p waves that may or may not have a fixed relationship to the QRS. The surface ECG usually reveals p waves with vectors different from the sinus node activation pattern (Figs. 5.6 and 5.7). Normal sinus rhythm presents with P waves that are positive in I,

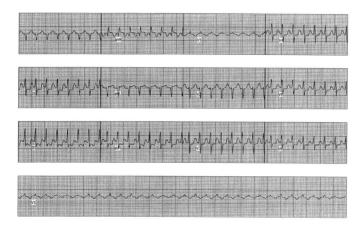

Fig. 5.6 Standard 12 lead ECG example of atrial tachycardia

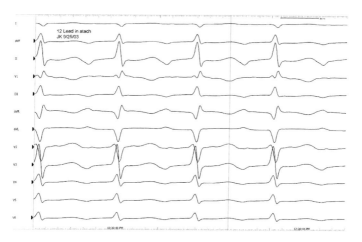

Fig. 5.7 Magnified 12 Lead to discern P wave activity

II, and negative in AVR. A tachycardia originating near the sinus node or from within the sinus tissue, it would appear similar to sinus activation pattern and the possibility of sinus node reentry should be considered. The atrial cycle length of atrial tachycardias are generally longer than atrial flutter cycle lengths that are often ~200-250 msec. The P wave morphology of atrial tachycardias often appear similar to sinus P waves versus peaked saw tooth pattern waves seen in atrial flutter. On occasion, we find that what appeared to be an atrial tachycardia on surface ECG was found to be an atypical atrial flutter during an EP study.

The mechanism may consist of a focal automaticity, intra-atrial reentry, or triggered automaticity. While focal automaticity is generally resistant to termination by burst pacing, reentry or triggered automaticity based tachycardias are often induced and terminated by burst pacing.

Atrial tachycardias may occur in children for a variety of reasons including congenital heart disease, particularly in the very young with decreasing prevalence with age. It may be seen in adults over time as a lone problem or accompanying myocarditis, thyroid disease, both acute and chronic pulmonary disease, and in patient with cardiomyopathies.

Clinical Presentation

Patient often present with a chief complaint of palpitations or 'skipping.' Their ECG may reveal rates that may be within the range of normal sinus rhythm or sinus tachycardia up to rates around 180 bpm. The intermediate rates may make it hard to discern between sinus or atrial tachycardia, though one would expect that the setting in which the ECG is obtained will improve the specificity. For example, sitting quietly in the office with sudden onset of tachycardia at 165 bpm 1:1 AV conduction would be more consistent with an atrial tachycardia than sinus tachycardia. However, these tachycardias present as persistent and stable rhythms at rates mimicking sinus tachycardia and difficult to discern without a 12 lead ECG. The differential diagnosis of underlying etiology requires a detailed patient history that may suggest an acute disease process such as pulmonary embolus, RV failure, thyroid disease, pulmonary disease.

Clinical Management

The treatment of underlying cause is naturally a first step for those patients in which direct trigger is found. However, the vast majority of patients will need to be treated with a tiered pharmacologic approach that may start with beta blockade or antiarrhythmic to control the frequency, duration, and symptoms associated with an atrial tachycardia while minimizing side effects from the drugs themselves. If there is a focal atrial morphology, then radiofrequency ablation of the site is a preferred strategy with a high probability of cure.

Electrophysiology Study and Ablation

Review of the 12 lead ECG often provides information regarding location and cycle length of the tachycardia. The consideration of location should be done prior to starting the procedure to avoid surprises and determine equipment that may be needed . The main consideration is whether the tachycardia is located in the left atrium or pulmonary veins which would require transeptal approach and anticoagulation. 3-D electro-anatomical and non-contact mapping is critical to localizing the circuit or focus while minimizing radiation exposure from fluoroscopy. There are several 3D mapping systems available which continuously improve their technology making mapping more efficient and accurate [9–11]. The approach to the EP study for atrial tachycardias assumes that single and 12 lead ECGs have been thoroughly reviewed with a differential diagnosis in place to help guide the strategy. During the EP study, one should consider the following:

1. Document baseline sinus rhythm, AH, HV intervals. Any pre-excitation? Is the AV conduction normal?
2. Select best leads to view P wave morphology on the EP recording system (Figs. 5.6 and 5.7)

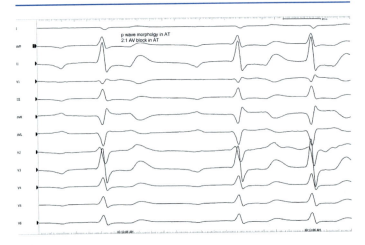

Fig. 5.8 2:1 block during atrial tachycardia confirm A-V dissociation ruling out AVRT

3. If in AT where does the 12 lead ECG localize the origin to?
4. 1:1 A-V conduction during tachycardia- Consider adenosine, and review baseline variable conduction or use ventricular burst pacing to separate A-V relationship ruling out AVRT (Figs. 5.8 and 5.9)
5. Attempt to determine mechanism: focal, triggered automaticity, or reentry . Use pacing maneuvers to attempt entrainment with concealed fusion to determine if a reentry mechanism is noted.
6. Characterize AV node function –Effective refractory periods using programmed stimulation should be done as part of any EP study
7. Any evidence of dual AV nodal physiology or accessory pathways?
8. 1:1 V-A conduction: Is it concentric? Is it decremental?
9. Add agents such as isoproterenol or atropine to alter autonomic tone to increase the probability of inducing SVT.

5 Diagnosis and Treatment of Supraventricular Tachycardias

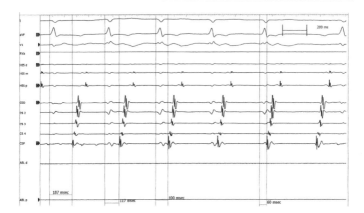

Fig. 5.9 Intracardiac recording confirming 12 lead of A-V dissociation during tachycardia. Note that the earliest atrial signal is located in the proximal coronary sinus electrode. This only narrows down location based on current electrodes. One can only say that the earliest atrial activation from the electrodes current in place is the proximal CS

10. Where is earliest atrial signal compared to surface P wave?
11. Consider phrenic nerve injury and confirm with pacing before ablating [12]

A patient may have an atrial tachycardia but may also develop other lab induced tachycardias including AVNRT, atrial fibrillation, or atrial flutter that may or may not have clinical significance.

The mapping of focal atrial tachycardias integrates electrogram analysis, timing, and is best done by utilizing 3D electroanatomical mapping systems to store geospatial points and minimize fluoroscopy. In focal atrial tachycardias, we often use a triggered mode screen format which provides a visual trigger on each atrial beat and allows us to map quickly obtaining the earliest atrial signal on the distal electrode of the ablation catheter compared to the surface P wave . Choosing the right reference on 3D

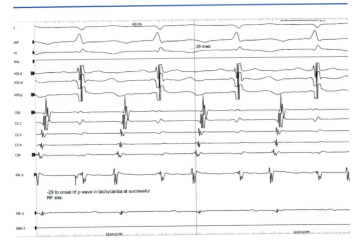

Fig. 5.10 EGM mapping of atrial tachycardia. Successful termination of the tachycardia was achieved using the earliest atrial signal is seen at the distal electrode of the ablation catheter (ABL d) at a location posterior to the coronary coronary sinus and 29 msec earlier than the onset of the surface P wave. It is directly under the Tricuspid valve – far field R waves can be seen

mapping is important. It is important to always consider that an early atrial endocardial signal in single chamber mapping, for example the right atrium, may be earliest on a 3D map of the right atrium but later than the surface P wave if the origin is in the left atrium, right superior pulmonary vein. The reference electrode chosen determines accuracy of origin as well as diagnosis when it comes to optimizing 3D mapping. There are various 3D mapping systems available. Figures 5.10 and 5.11 demonstrate EGM mapping of an atrial tachycardia localized to a site posterior to the coronary sinus os.

5 Diagnosis and Treatment of Supraventricular Tachycardias

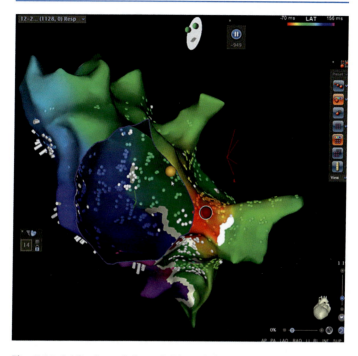

Fig. 5.11 LAO view of Carto 3 Map of the right atrium and earliest EGM. The site of ablation is denoted by dark red point

SVT Mapping Considerations

Different 3D mapping strategies will be utilized depending on the diagnosis of the SVT.

AVNRT In most cases, AVNRT 3D mapping will be only anatomical. Some operators may prefer to collect an entire right atrial anatomical geometry, marking out the tricuspid valve in detail. Others may choose to simply mark important anatomical sites with location tags and not collect the actual chamber. In either case, the most important anatomical marker in AVNRT mapping is a detailed His bundle, to prevent AV block. Marking the CS ostium is also helpful for safety. If multiple ablations are required to eliminate the slow pathway, it is helpful to use a different color tag to mark the site of effective ablation and places where multiple junctional beats were observed. In the event of a recovery of the slow pathway during the post-ablation testing phase, the electrophysiologist will be able to easy navigate back to the spot in question. Due to the sensitivity of the structures in the triangle of Koch, it is also recommended to use respiratory gating technology on the 3D map, and to take all anatomical tags consistently at end expiration. (Respirations can account for up to 5 mm of inaccuracy in 3D maps, and 5 mm can make a critical difference when trying to avoid AV block.)

AVRT Mapping a pathway can be done in multiple ways. In its simplest form, the 3D mapper can simply use location tags to mark areas of interest (AV fusion, AP potentials), so that the EP can return to those locations after exploring the entire valve. Electroanatomic (EA) mapping can also be beneficial. Window of interest choices must be made in order to properly map. It is usually best to map accessory pathways while pacing. If the pathway conducts both antegradely and retrogradely, pacing from either chamber will work; if the pathway only conducts retrogradely, you must pace from the ventricle. It is usually best to use the pacing spike of the catheter you are pacing as the "time zero" reference, and then map to the distal chamber (e.g., use RV catheter for reference while RV pacing, and annotate on atrial electrograms). When mapping this way, note that all times will be positive (no negative window). Therefore, a window of interest will usually be set at +20 to +150. A newer mapping strategy has recently been utilized for mapping AVRT. Advanced mapping technologies have allowed for better annotation of local vs. farfield signals, allowing the mapping window to be left open to include both atrial and ventricular signals. This "open window mapping" strategy relies additionally on an "extended early-meets-late" algorithm that identifies lines of block. The location of the accessory pathway, then, would be a break in this line of block. Figure 5.11 shows a mid-septal break in the "line of block" (which is the tricuspid annulus), clearly locating the pathway away lower than the Bundle of His. See Chap. 4 on WPW for more on mapping AVRT.

Atrial Tachycardia Atrial tachycardias can be surprisingly difficult to map. Challenges include previous ablations (AT is often present post AF ablation; see AF chapter for more on post-AF LA AT), areas of scar, multiple tachycardias (or multifocal AT), varying cycle lengths, and difficulty inducing and sustaining AT. Sometimes differentiating mechanism (automatic, trigger, microreentry, or macroreentry) can be problematic. Mapping reentrant atrial tachycardias is covered in the atrial flutter chapter. But because triggered activity and microreentry can mask as macroreentry, we recommend approaching the mapping for AT in the same way as mapping a macroreentrant tachycardia. By using the DePonti algorithm for calculating the window of interest, focal, microreentrant, and macroreentrant possibilities will all be taken into account during the EA 3D mapping. If reentry has been entirely ruled out by pacing maneuvers, the window can simply be set to have the backwards interval timed at 80–100 ms before p wave onset. If p waves cannot be observed, it is best to administer adenosine to set a window. The window of interest's relationship to the p wave is critical to accurately mapping the AT.

It is important to recognize that no matter how high density and rapid the mapping system may be, 3D mapping will be impossible with multifocal AT and extremely difficult with rapidly changing ATs. Due to the limitations of color-based window-of-interest mapping, some ATs with complex mechanisms (microreentry in scar) will need more advanced mapping algorithms to determine mechanism. In the case below, traditional mapping located a focal breakout on the RA posterolateral wall (Fig. 5.12), but ablation was unsuccessful. EGMs in an adjacent area of scar had been excluded by the window of interest and produced confusing results with included (Figs. 5.13 and 5.14). An advanced

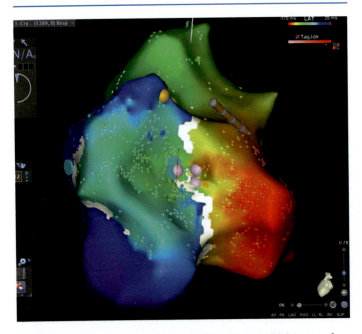

Fig. 5.12 Open Window Mapping on the Carto 3 system. Pink tags are fractionated (fused A and V) EGMs. Yellow tags are Bundle of His

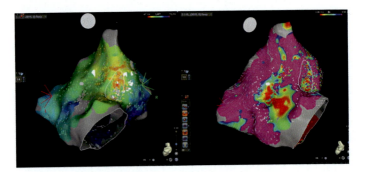

Fig. 5.13 LAT early at RA posterolateral site

5 Diagnosis and Treatment of Supraventricular Tachycardias

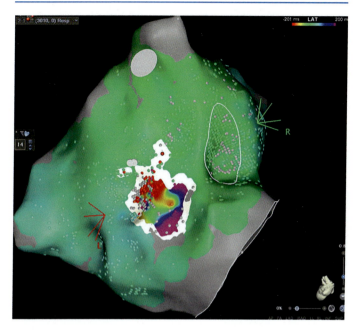

Fig. 5.14 Annotation of double potentials in scar with traditional mapping provides confusing picture of arrhythmia mechanism

mapping algorithm called Coherent (Biosense Webster, Carto 3) was able to determine the Small circuit reentry through scar, resulting in successful ablation (Fig. 5.15).

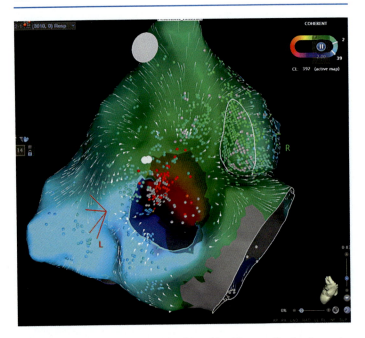

Fig. 5.15 Coherent mapping Algorithm identifies small circuit reentry through scar

References

1. Suenari KJ, et al. Gender differences in the clinical characteristics and atrioventricular nodal conduction properties in patients with atrioventricular nodal reentrant tachycardia. Cardiovasc Electrophysiol. 2010;21(10):1114–9.
2. Walfridsson, et al. Wolff-Parkinson-White syndrome and atrioventricular nodal re-entry tachycardia in a Swedish population: consequences on health-related quality of life. Pacing Clin Electrophysiol. 2009;32(10):1299–306.
3. Jackman WM, et al. Treatment of supraventricular tachycardia due to atrioventricular nodal reentry, by radiofrequency catheter ablation of slow-pathway conduction. N Engl J Med. 1992;327(5):313–8.
4. Stabile G, et al. The predictive value of junctional beats during the radio-frequency transcatheter ablation of the slow pathway of the nodal reentry circuit. Ital Cardiol. 1999;29(5):549–54.

5. Demosthenes GK, et al. Atrioventricular nodal Reentrant tachycardia. Circulation. 2010;122:831–40.
6. Demosthenes GK, et al. Classification of electrophysiological types of atrioventricular nodal re-entrant tachycardia: a reappraisal. Europace. 2013;15:1231–40.
7. Reddy V, et al. Para-Hisian entrainment: a novel pacing maneuver to differentiate orthodromic atrioventricular reentrant tachycardia from atrioventricular nodal reentrant tachycardia. J Cardiovasc Electrophysiol. 2003;14(12):1321–8.
8. Hiaro, et al. Para-Hisian pacing. Circulation. 1996;94(5):1027–35.
9. Wu RC, Berger R, Calkins H. Catheter ablation of atrial flutter and macroreentrant atrial tachycardia. Curr Opin Cardiol. 2002;17(1):58–64.
10. Chen SA, Chiang CE, Yang CJ, et al. Sustained atrial tachycardia in adult patients. Electrophysiological characteristics, pharmacological response, possible mechanisms, and effects of radiofrequency ablation. Circulation. 1994;90(3):1262–78.
11. Marcus W, et al. Catheter ablation of non-sustained focal right atrial tachycardia guided by virtual non-contact electrograms. Europace. 2011;13:876–82.
12. Huemer M, et al. Mapping of the left-sided phrenic nerve course in patients undergoing left atrial catheter ablations. Pacing Clin Electrophysiol. 2014;

Wolff-Parkinson-White (WPW) Syndrome

Jeffrey M. Vinocur

Abstract

The bidirectional accessory pathways that typically cause WPW can have a variety of manifestations. Orthodromic AVRT is the most common, and is similar to other forms of SVT. Uncommon manifestations include antidromic AVRT, bystander pathway conduction during other arrhythmias (atrial arrhythmias, AVNRT), and dyssynchrony-induced cardiomyopathy. Although rare, the most serious manifestation of WPW is sudden death, due to atrial fibrillation with rapid conduction down the pathway. Sudden death can occur even in completely asymptomatic patients; therefore this risk should be carefully considered any time WPW is diagnosed. Specific recommendations for risk stratification in children and young adults with asymptomatic WPW have been published.

J. M. Vinocur (✉)
Department of Pediatrics, Yale University School of Medicine,
New Haven, CT, USA
e-mail: jeffrey.vinocur@yale.edu

© The Author(s), under exclusive license to Springer Nature Switzerland AG 2023
D. T. Huang et al. (eds.), *Cardiac Electrophysiology in Clinical Practice*, In Clinical Practice,
https://doi.org/10.1007/978-3-031-41479-4_6

Pharmacologic therapy for SVT can include beta-blockers and class I or III anti-arrhythmics Digoxin and calcium-channel blockers are contraindicated. Catheter ablation is frequently recommended for patients with SVT (especially if other features, such as syncope, preexcited atrial fibrillation, or antidromic AVRT are present), and increasingly recommended for asymptomatic patients depending on the results of risk stratification.

Multiple mapping strategies can be employed, including earliest atrial activation (in ventricular pacing or orthodromic AVRT) and earliest ventricular pacing (in sinus rhythm or atrial pacing). Each has strengths and weaknesses with regard to electrogram clarity, catheter stability, potential for misleading fusion, and ability to detect AV node injury during ablation. Ideally, 3D mapping is used. Standard tip radiofrequency (or cryo) ablation generally suffices, often early in the first lesion, if applied to a carefully mapped and selected location.

Keywords

Wolff-Parkinson-White Syndrome · Ventricular preexcitation · Orthodromic tachycardia · Supraventricular tachycardia · Preexcited atrial fibrillation · Catheter ablation

WPW, in its full form, is the combination of ventricular preexcitation on ECG plus palpitations (due to orthodromic AVRT). Often the term "Asymptomatic WPW" is used, somewhat confusingly, to refer to the finding of a WPW-type baseline ECG without any subjective or documented arrhythmia. In either case, the electrical substrate is that of an accessory AV pathway with antegrade (and almost always retrograde) conduction.

These pathways can support several arrhythmias (orthodromic AVRT, antidromic AVRT, and pathway-to-pathway reentry in patients with multiple pathways), and act as bystanders to others (most often atrial arrhythmias, although AVNRT with bystander pathway conduction can occur). Paroxysmal SVT from orthodromic AVRT is by far the most common manifestation. However, special attention must be drawn to the entity of atrial fibrillation with "bystander" conduction down the accessory pathway, because this can lead to sudden death, even in previously asymp-

6 Wolff-Parkinson-White (WPW) Syndrome

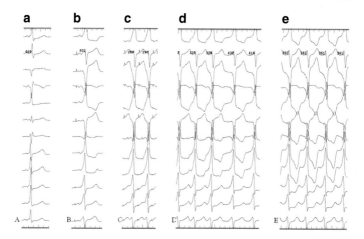

Fig. 6.1 Surface ECG morphologies from a patient with WPW in different situations. (**a**) Sinus rhythm with subtle preexcitation, (**b**) Preexcitation maximized by slow atrial pacing plus adenosine, (**c**) Preexcitation maximized by rapid atrial pacing, (**d**) Irregular rhythm with variable degrees of preexcitation due to atrial fibrillation, (**e**) Regular rhythm with maximal preexcitation due to antidromic AVRT

tomatic persons. Finally, left ventricular systolic dysfunction, i.e. dyssynchrony-induced cardiomyopathy, usually related to pathways on the anterior tricuspid annulus, is a non-arrhythmic manifestation of WPW.

Orthodromic AVRT in the setting of WPW is comparable to AVRT caused by concealed accessory pathways, as described elsewhere. Antidromic AVRT is an uncommon wide-complex tachycardia using the accessory pathway antegrade and the AV node retrograde (see Fig. 6.1e). It is one of several so-called "preexcited tachycardias," a category that also includes preexcited atrial fibrillation (see Fig. 6.1d) and almost every other form of SVT with bystander accessory pathway conduction (this can occur with AVNRT, atrial tachycardia, etc).

The diagnosis of WPW is generally straightforward from the baseline ECG. Occasionally fusion between sinus and ventricular beats falsely gives the appearance of preexcitation (for example, late-coupled ventricular bigeminy can look like preexcitation alternans). Preexcitation can sometime be subtle (see Figs. 6.1a and 6.2),

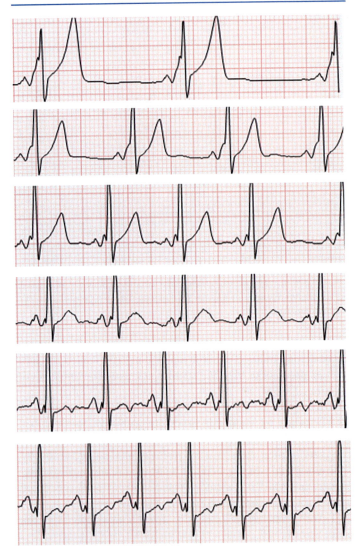

Fig. 6.2 Series of strips from a single patient at various sinus rates, demonstrating variable degrees of fusion (related to autonomic effects on AV node conduction time, with antegrade pathway conduction present throughout); this type of "loss of preexcitation at faster heart rates" does not indicate *anything* about a pathway being "low-risk"

due to variable degrees of fusion between antegrade nodal and antegrade pathway conduction. Subtle preexcitation is more likely when atrial depolarization reaches the pathway late (i.e. left-sided pathways), when nodal conduction is relatively rapid (i.e. young patient, elevated sympathetic tone), or when pathway conduction velocity is slow (certain types of atypical pathways, discussed elsewhere). Antegrade pathway conduction can be absent or intermittent above certain atrial rates, depending on the pathway's refractory period. Antegrade pathway conduction can also be absent for reasons unrelated to pathway refractoriness (so-called "latent" pathways), including the phenomenon of concealed penetration of the His-Purkinje wavefront retrograde into the pathway (see Fig. 6.3a).

Additional rhythm recording (Holter, event recorder) may be indicated depending on symptoms. Echocardiography is indicated at baseline (to evaluate for comorbid structural heart disease,

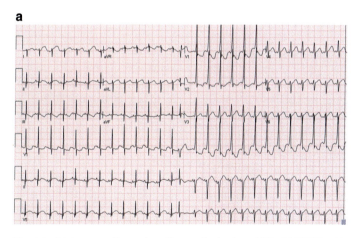

Fig. 6.3 (**a**) Apparent "intermittent" preexcitation in a child with WPW, with narrow QRS due to repetitive concealed penetration of the His-Purkinje wavefront retrograde into the pathway, until a PAC disturbs the pattern and allows antegrade pathway conduction at the same sinus rate; this patient had "high-risk features" demonstrated at EP study. (**b**) Truly intermittent preexcitation (on a beat-by-beat basis) in a different patient with WPW and hypertrophic cardiomyopathy; note half-scale voltage for precordial leads

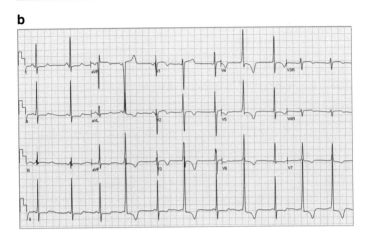

Fig. 6.3 (continued)

including Ebstein anomaly of the tricuspid valve, other forms of congenital heart disease, and hypertrophic cardiomyopathy) and perhaps periodically thereafter (to evaluate for ventricular dysfunction). Family screening is not generally recommended, as the recurrence risk in relatives is only modestly elevated (although certainly families with multiple affected members do occur).

Finally, the risk for sudden death must be considered. The mechanism of sudden death is believed to be that of rapidly conducted atrial fibrillation resulting in rapid irregular ventricular stimulation and eventually ventricular fibrillation (see Fig. 6.4). Patients with WPW are at increased risk for atrial fibrillation, even in the absence of structural heart disease. Therefore the risk of sudden death depends primarily on the antegrade conduction characteristics of the pathway. Patients with syncope, documented preexcited atrial fibrillation, multiple preexcited morphologies (since multiple pathways may alternate to allow rapid ventricular stimulation), and SVT (especially antidromic SVT) are at increased risk. Generally, older patients are believed to be at decreased risk, presumably because of survivor bias.

A 2012 consensus statement from PACES (the Pediatric and Congenital EP Society) and HRS (the Heart Rhythm Society) pro-

6 Wolff-Parkinson-White (WPW) Syndrome

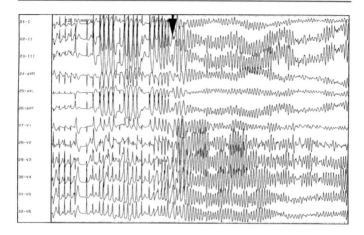

Fig. 6.4 Preexcited atrial fibrillation may degenerate into ventricular fibrillation (reproduced with permission [2])

vided guidance for the management of asymptomatic WPW in children and young adults [1]. Although studies differ about the exact magnitude of the risk for sudden death (e.g. between 0.1 and 5 per 1000 patient-years), the guideline authors provided class IIa recommendations for risk stratification using a staged approach with non-invasive and often invasive testing (see Figs. 6.5, 6.6, and 6.7), followed by varying recommendations for ablation depending on the findings (see Fig. 6.8, left panel).

Recent data have called into question the entire paradigm of risk stratification. Although there is statistical correlation between pathway behavior and risk, a large multi-center study showed antegrade conduction properties (and/or presence of symptoms) to have poor discriminative ability for identifying any reasonable subset with a truly low risk of life-threatening event (see Fig. 6.9). Another study from the same dataset showed that the finding of intermittent preexcitation did not correlate reliably to pathway characteristics.

As a result, current thinking and clinical practice has shifted towards a default strategy of catheter ablation for most patients with WPW, excepting perhaps those with elevated risk for complication due to proximity to the compact AV node, especially if

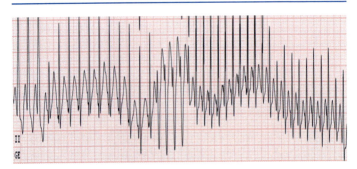

Fig. 6.5 Strip from a patient with WPW undergoing exercise stress test. Preexcitation was present for the majority of the test, up through the first 3 beats on this strip. Then there is abrupt loss of preexcitation (in a single beat, associated with clear increase in PR) in the setting of sinus tachycardia to just over 200 bpm; this is the sort of abrupt loss that was considered low-risk behavior under the traditional approach to risk stratification. After 11 beats of sinus tachycardia with antegrade nodal conduction, SVT begins, at a rate of nearly 300 bpm, with rate-related aberrancy for the first 4 beats

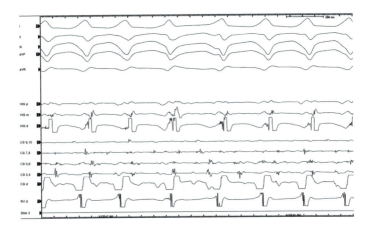

Fig. 6.6 Atrial fibrillation with rapid antegrade pathway conduction; the shortest preexcited RR interval (SPERRI) was 212 ms when AF was induced intentionally at EP study for evaluation of pathway behavior

cryoablation is not available. The newer data have been incorporated into a proposed modification of the older guideline flowchart (see Fig. 6.8).

6 Wolff-Parkinson-White (WPW) Syndrome

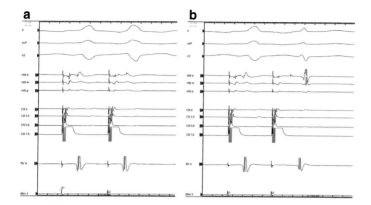

Fig. 6.7 Surface and intracardiac electrograms from atrial extrastimuli testing showing the accessory pathway effective refractory period with drive train S1 cycle length 400 ms and (**a**) S2 = 300 ms resulting in simultaneous antegrade pathway and nodal conduction with H-V interval < 0, compared to (**b**) S2 = 290 ms resulting in exclusively nodal conduction, with a much longer PR interval, normal H-V interval, and narrow QRS

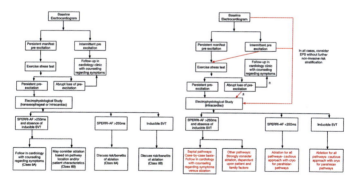

Fig. 6.8 Comparison of flowcharts from 2012 PACES/HRS guidelines for risk stratification of asymptomatic children and young adults with WPW with a proposed approach based on emerging data (reprinted with permission [3]). SPERRI-AF: shortest preexcited R-R interval in atrial fibrillation

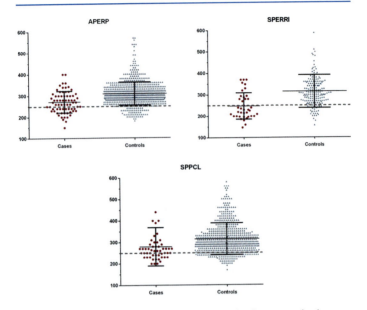

Fig. 6.9 Comparison of antegrade pathway conduction properties between cases with life-threatening arrhythmia (cardiac arrest, sudden death, or rapid preexcited atrial fibrillation) and controls, demonstrating the poor sensitivity of the traditional 250 ms cutoff as well as substantial between-group overlap limiting utility of any specific cutoff (reprinted with permission [4]). APERP: accessory pathway effective refractory period, SPERRI: shortest preexcited R-R interval (in AF), SPPCL: shortest preexcited paced cycle length (during decremental atrial pacing)

Management

Pharmacologic

For patients with WPW, medication is generally reserved for management of SVT (orthodromic AVRT) in patients felt not to be at high risk for sudden death or who decline ablation. As AVRT is itself a predictor of elevated risk (perhaps because rapid atrial activation during SVT can promote atrial fibrillation), ablation is routinely recommended for patients with WPW and SVT.

For management of AVRT, unlike in patients with concealed accessory pathways, digoxin and calcium-channel blockers are considered contraindicated in patients with WPW due to an association with sudden death (AV node blockade is felt to promote antegrade conduction down the pathway). Although the same concern theoretically exists for beta-blockers, these medications have been used extensively in patients with WPW without convincing evidence for untoward effects. However, it is important to realize that beta-blockade does not reliably protect against rapidly conducted atrial fibrillation and sudden death in predisposed patients. Therefore, beta-blockers are primarily appropriate for management of SVT in patients not felt to be at high risk for malignant arrhythmia.

Anti-arrhythmic agents with direct pathway activity (class I and perhaps class III agents) are also effective for treatment of AVRT, and are frequently used when beta-blockers are unsuccessful or undesirable because of concern about malignant arrhythmia risk.

Similar principles apply regarding acute management of patients with WPW. For patients in AVRT, certainly intravenous calcium-channel blockers should be avoided. Adenosine and beta-blockers are reasonable, although appropriate resuscitation equipment should be available with adenosine due to its tendency to induce atrial fibrillation that could be rapidly conducted. Channel-active intravenous anti-arrhythmic medications can also be used, depending on local availability. When patients present in preexcited atrial fibrillation, emergent intervention is required, even if the rhythm is hemodynamically well tolerated. Immediate sedated cardioversion is prudent. Any delay (while awaiting NPO status, pharmacologic cardioversion, or EP lab activation) can be considered only in a closely-monitored setting with full resuscitation equipment immediately available.

Catheter-Based

Mapping

There are numerous approaches to mapping WPW, which offers flexibility to change strategies if needed. It is important to understand that no one approach will always be optimal; the choice should be individualized based on patient- and equipment-specific factors.

All of the standard approaches for typical accessory pathways involve activation mapping around the tricuspid or mitral annulus, ideally with 3D mapping (which has been shown in some studies to improve success rates and can minimize or eliminate radiation exposure from fluoroscopy). Mapping can target the earliest atrial activation in any rhythm using the pathway retrograde (orthodromic AVRT, ventricular pacing) or earliest ventricular activation in any rhythm using the pathway antegrade (sinus, atrial pacing, antidromic AVRT). Each approach has its strengths and weaknesses, particularly because mapping and ablation should generally be performed in the same rhythm, leading to tradeoffs between facilitating mapping and facilitating safe and effective ablation (see Table 6.1).

Table 6.1 Overview of the relative advantages of the various mapping approaches in WPW. In some situations, difficulties can be reduced by the techniques described in the text, indicated by +/++ or +/+++ in the table

Mapping target	Earliest A	Earliest A	Earliest V	Earliest V	Earliest V
Rhythm	Ortho-AVRT	V pacing	Sinus	A pacing	Anti-AVRT
Unambiguous map (no pathway/node fusion)	+++	+/++	+	+/++	+++
Crisp V electrograms (His-Purkinje activation)	++	+	+	+	+
Ability to assess AV node during ablation	+++	+	+/+++	+/+++	+
Stable catheter position during ablation	+/++	++	+++	+++	+

One of the biggest pitfalls with mapping in WPW is the possibility of fusion between pathway and nodal conduction, which can occur when mapping in sinus, atrial paced, and ventricular paced rhythms. This can be partially avoided by carefully adjusting the rhythm to promote pathway conduction, for example by accelerating the pacing rate, changing the pacing site to be closer to the pathway (best demonstrated by comparing the degree of preexcitation in right vs left atrial pacing at the same cycle length), or even administering medication (e.g. phenylephrine) to slow AV nodal conduction. Mapping in AVRT completely eliminates this concern. Mapping in orthodromic AVRT provides an additional advantage of crisper ventricular electrograms (due to His-Purkinje activation), sometimes resulting in more easily interpreted signals. Alternatively, differential pacing from either side of the pathway can be performed so that the electrical wavefront is from the opposite direction from the presumed path of a slanted pathway. This technique separates the local electrogram components resulting in easier interpretation of electrograms and the resulting map. This approach is also reported to often unmask accessory pathway potentials, which are appealing targets for ablation.

Regardless of mapping strategy, it is critical to target the absolute earliest electrogram in the targeted chamber relative to a fixed reference point such as a coronary sinus bipole (for retrograde mapping) or a surface lead with a clearly identifiable deflection (for antegrade mapping). Although tempting, it can be quite misleading to target sites with short local A-V interval (for antegrade mapping) or V-A interval (for retrograde mapping); while this local "fusion" is frequently present at successful sites (see Figs. 6.10, 6.11c, 6.12b, 6.13c, 6.14a, 6.15, 6.16a), it can also be present at distant sites where both components of the local electrogram are delayed to similar degrees. Similar to mapping PVCs, the relevance of a suspected site can be confirmed independent of the relative timing data by analyzing precocity relative to surface QRS onset, and local unipolar electrogram timing and morphology.

Because almost all pathways are direct AV connections crossing the mitral or tricuspid annulus, interpretation of the maps is usually straightforward, with the earliest area being a point (or a

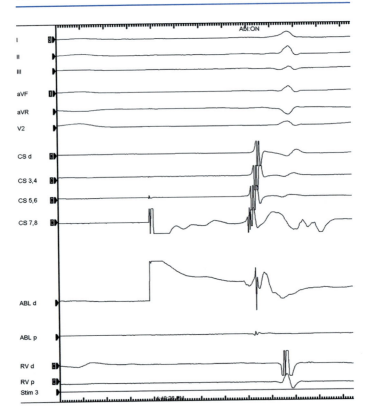

Fig. 6.10 Surface and intracardiac electrograms at the site of successful ablation from mapping earliest ventricular activation in sinus rhythm, note the very early ventricular component recorded from the ablation catheter. Artifact in CS7,8 and ABLd channels relates to onset of RF delivery

Fig. 6.11 (a) Right atrial activation map (RAO and LAO/cranial views) of earliest atrial activation in AVRT of the patient in Fig. 6.8 with an anteroseptal pathway. Yellow markers indicate sites where His potential was recorded; white/pink coloration indicates the area of earliest activation; blue markers indicate site of successful cryoablation. (b) Corresponding fluoroscopy (RAO and LAO views) of catheter positions at the successful site. (c) Electrograms from the surface ECG, His, coronary sinus, right ventricle, and ablation catheter at the successful site

6 Wolff-Parkinson-White (WPW) Syndrome 117

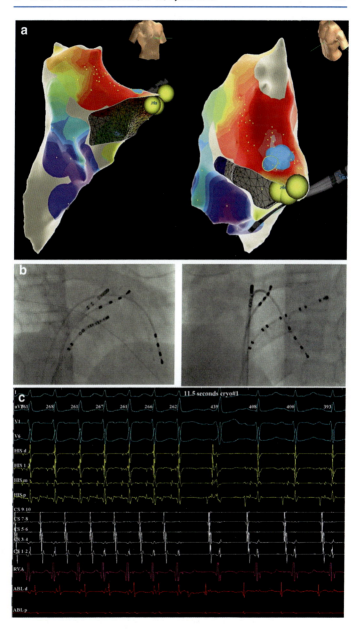

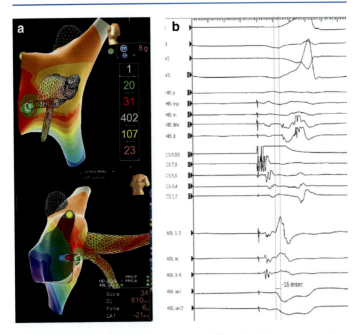

Fig. 6.12 (**a**) Right atrial activation map (LPO and LAO views) of earliest ventricular activation in atrial pacing of a patient with a right posteroseptal pathway. White/pink coloration indicates the area of earliest activation. (**b**) Electrograms from the surface ECG, His catheter, coronary sinus catheter, and roving/ablation catheter at the site indicated by the green marker. Although only 16 msec prior to QRS onset, early activation was well bracketed and unipolar tip recording showed a QS morphology. Ablation at this site eliminated the pathway within 1 s

small line running across the atrioventricular groove), and with progressively later points to either side along the annulus (see Figs. 6.11a, 6.12a, 6.13a, b). A broad area of earliest electrograms suggests (1) imprecise electrogram interpretation that may benefit from careful manual review or switch to a different mapping strategy, (2) fusion between pathway and nodal conduction if plausible in the rhythm being used, (3) fusion between multiple pathways, and/or (4) that the true earliest area has not been

6 Wolff-Parkinson-White (WPW) Syndrome

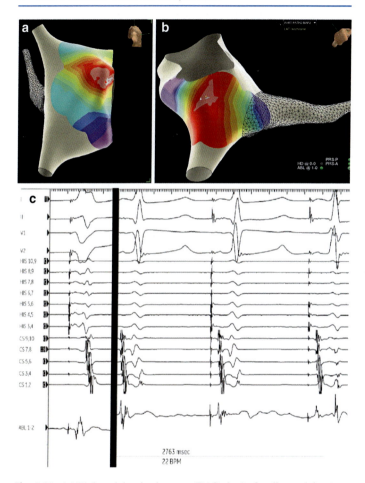

Fig. 6.13 (**a**) Right atrial activation map (RAO view) of earliest atrial activation during ventricular pacing of a patient with WPW and two bidirectional accessory pathways. The right anterolateral pathway's antegrade conduction was weak and prone to mechanical suppression but retrograde conduction was readily mapped after change in strategy. (**b**) Right atrial activation map (LAO/caudal view) of earliest atrial activation during orthodromic AVRT in the same patient. Antegrade conduction was not readily mapped due to complex difficult-to-annotate electrograms through a large portion of the posterior annulus, but retrograde conduction was readily mapped after change in strategy. (**c**) Electrograms from the same patient. First beat, site where ablation eliminated the anterolateral pathway within 1 s. Remaining beats, site where ablation eliminated the posterior pathway within 3 s

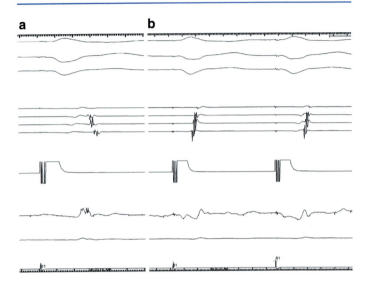

Fig. 6.14 Surface and intracardiac electrograms (**a**) before and (**b**) just after successful ablation performed during ventricular pacing in a patient with WPW via a left lateral accessory pathway. Note the change from eccentric retrograde conduction (coronary sinus activation distal to proximal) to absent retrograde conduction exposing V-A dissociated sinus rhythm. Displayed channels are as in Fig. 6.15

explored, for example on the opposite side of the atrial septum, or (rarely) within an atrial appendage or coronary sinus.

Entrainment

Although WPW supports SVT via a reentrant mechanism, it can be mapped like a focal tachycardia by following the activation pattern towards the earliest site, which should correspond to where the pathway crosses the atrioventricular groove. Thus, entrainment maneuvers are not critical to mapping of WPW. However, they can occasionally be useful diagnostically (e.g. in evaluating whether an SVT is AVRT) or when there is uncertainty about whether the pathway is left-sided or right-sided (although usually this is evident from the retrograde atrial activa-

6 Wolff-Parkinson-White (WPW) Syndrome

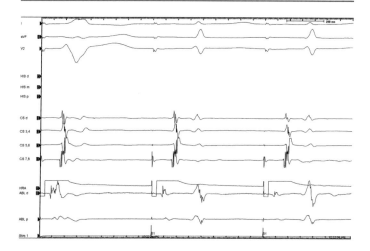

Fig. 6.15 Surface and intracardiac electrograms showing loss of preexcitation (between first and second beats) due to ablation performed during atrial pacing in a patient with WPW. Note the very early local ventricular activation recorded from the ablation catheter on the first beat, compared to the well-separated atrial and ventricular electrograms on the later beats

tion sequencing, see Fig. 6.17). When performed, the maneuvers are comparable to those used for AVRT.

Ablation

Correct, precise mapping is the cornerstone of successful WPW ablation. Most pathways are delicate and can be easily eliminated with energy delivery at the correct location. However, there are important considerations with regard to the rhythm in which ablation is performed (see Table 6.1). Because cardiac filling can vary with heart rate and A-V relationship, the exact location of the pathway may differ in different rhythms and therefore mapping and ablation are ideally performed in the same rhythm.

Catheter stability can be an issue with abrupt rhythm changes at the moment of ablation success, such as when AVRT breaks to sinus rhythm with elimination of pathway conduction. This difficulty can be minimized by mapping in AVRT and then ablating in V-entrained AVRT. By carefully entraining just slightly faster

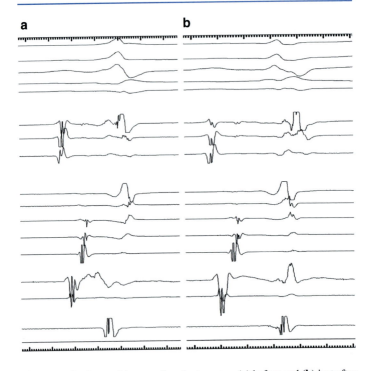

Fig. 6.16 Surface and intracardiac electrograms (**a**) before and (**b**) just after successful ablation performed during sinus rhythm in a patient with WPW. Note again the very early local ventricular activation recorded from the ablation catheter during preexcitation, compared to the well-separated atrial and ventricular electrograms during nodal conduction. Unlike the previous figure, this patient has relatively subtle preexcitation so the changes in surface PR interval and coronary sinus AV interval are less prominent than the local change at the ablation site. Displayed channels are as in Fig. 6.15

than the tachycardia (often achieving sustained fusion in QRS morphology), the map remains accurate, but at the time of pathway success there is only a small change in hemodynamics (from fused tachycardia to fully paced tachycardia) and thus less chance of catheter dislodgement. However, this precludes the possibility of monitoring antegrade AV node function during ablation. Conversely, catheter stability is less likely to be an issue when

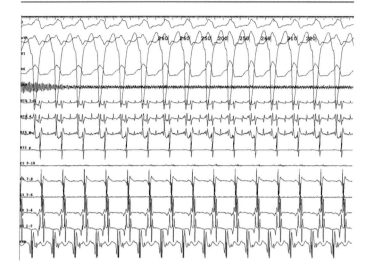

Fig. 6.17 Orthodromic AVRT with LBBB aberrancy and earliest atrial activation at the His position, in a patient with an anteroseptal pathway

ablating in sinus or paced rhythm, except in the situation of V paced rhythm with no retrograde nodal conduction, when V-A dissociation can result in cannon A waves and intermittent sinus capture beats. In this situation, quickly switching to simultaneous V and A pacing can improve stability. Finally, when stability is a persistent issue, cryoablation (with its ability to adhere to tissue) can be helpful even if far from the normal conduction system. Force-sensing catheters and intracardiac echo can both be helpful in determining whether stability and contact are appropriate, particularly in challenging locations such as the right free wall.

When ablating near the AV node, antegrade properties of the normal conduction system should be continuously monitored. This is easy in orthodromic AVRT (see Fig. 6.11c) as antegrade conduction is exposed during both SVT and sinus rhythm after successful termination. However, it is impossible during ventricular pacing (including V-entrained AVRT), except by alternating between V pacing and A pacing in an attempt to monitor both antegrade nodal and retrograde pathway conduction (a technique that is much easier and safer with cryoablation, due to catheter adherence and reversibility of effect). The normal conduction system can also usually be assessed during sinus or atrial paced rhythm, as elimination of both nodal and pathway conduction results in AV block, and elimination of nodal conduction alone results in QRS widening (maximal preexcitation). However, when preexcitation is maximal at baseline (due to rapid atrial pacing, see Fig. 6.1c, or when nodal conduction times are long or the pacing site is much nearer to pathway than node), it is possible to injure the normal conduction without any outward sign. Unfortunately, this results in a tradeoff between optimal mapping, in which maximal preexcitation is helpful, and safest ablation, where fused conduction is required.

Once a mapping strategy has been chosen and executed, an appropriate site identified, and an ablation strategy selected, the catheter is carefully positioned and energy is delivered. It is important to anticipate which aspects of the rhythm need to be monitored during ablation to assess effect and, potentially, AV node conduction); usually success is obvious (see Figs. 6.14 and 6.15) but occasionally it can be fairly subtle (see Fig. 6.16). At an optimal site, pathway conduction can frequently be eliminated within a second or two of RF delivery. Ongoing ablation (beyond 5 or at most 10 s) should be avoided at ineffective sites; although "success" will sometimes be achieved late, this is often due to partial heating from the periphery of the lesion, increasing the risk of early recurrence either later in lesion delivery or immediately after energy delivery is completed. Additionally, these lesions can result in tissue edema and local electrogram fragmentation, both of which can interfere with subsequent mapping and ablation.

Usually, careful adjustment of the targeted site (with further mapping using the same or a different strategy, if necessary) will ultimately result in a rapidly successful lesion. For the same reasons, large tip or irrigated RF should rarely be required, except perhaps when delivered power is temperature-limited to only a few watts (a situation occasionally encountered with right posteroseptal pathways). Most pathways with early coronary sinus activation can be more safely ablated from within the left atrium, but occasional pathways are truly best targeted in the coronary venous system (particularly the middle cardiac vein), being aware of the risk of coronary artery injury in these locations.

After ablation, a complete EP study should be repeated to document absence of any additional arrhythmia substrate or (if relevant) AV node injury. Of note, patients that had preexcited atrial fibrillation do not necessarily require therapy beyond accessory pathway ablation (which seems to reduce the atrial fibrillation substrate), unless ongoing atrial fibrillation is anticipated due to age or comorbidity. Adenosine bolus can sometimes unmask residual pathway conduction, and is reasonable as a routine part of the post-ablation study, but is particularly helpful when pathway conduction is absent due to mechanical trauma or edema from an imperfectly targeted ablation attempt. Post-ablation repolarization abnormalities, including T wave inversion and QT prolongation, are quite common after WPW ablation and attributed to "T wave memory" or "cardiac memory" (see Fig. 6.18); frank ST depression or elevation is less common and should prompt consideration of coronary artery injury. A 30- to 60-minute waiting period is prudent due to the chance of early recurrence.

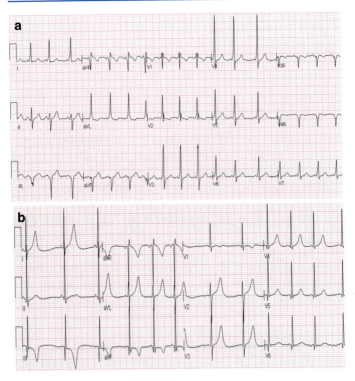

Fig. 6.18 (a) Baseline ECG of a patient with WPW due to a middle cardiac vein pathway. Despite the subtle difference in preexcitation on the first beat, the patient had only one pathway. (b) Same patient immediately after ablation, demonstrating repolarization abnormalities consistent with the "T wave memory" phenomenon

References

1. Pediatric and Congenital Electrophysiology Society (PACES), Heart Rhythm Society (HRS), American College of Cardiology Foundation (ACCF), American Heart Association (AHA), American Academy of Pediatrics (AAP), Canadian Heart Rhythm Society (CHRS), Cohen MI, Triedman JK, Cannon BC, Davis AM, Drago F, Janousek J, Klein GJ, Law IH, Morady FJ, Paul T, Perry JC, Sanatani S, Tanel RE. PACES/HRS expert consensus statement on the management of the asymptomatic

young patient with a Wolff-Parkinson-White (WPW, ventricular preexcitation) electrocardiographic pattern: developed in partnership between the Pediatric and Congenital Electrophysiology Society (PACES) and the Heart Rhythm Society (HRS). Endorsed by the governing bodies of PACES, HRS, the American College of Cardiology Foundation (ACCF), the American Heart Association (AHA), the American Academy of Pediatrics (AAP), and the Canadian Heart Rhythm Society (CHRS). Heart Rhythm. 2012;9(6):1006–24.
2. Delise P, Sciarra L. Sudden cardiac death in patients with ventricular preexcitation. Card Electrophysiol Clin. 2020;12(4):519–25.
3. Chubb H, Ceresnak SR. A proposed approach to the asymptomatic pediatric patient with Wolff-Parkinson-White pattern. HeartRhythm Case Rep. 2020;6(1):2–7.
4. Etheridge SP, Escudero CA, Blaufox AD, Law IH, Dechert-Crooks BE, Stephenson EA, Dubin AM, Ceresnak SR, Motonaga KS, Skinner JR, Marcondes LD, Perry JC, Collins KK, Seslar SP, Cabrera M, Uzun O, Cannon BC, Aziz PF, Kubuš P, Tanel RE, Valdes SO, Sami S, Kertesz NJ, Maldonado J, Erickson C, Moore JP, Asakai H, Mill L, Abcede M, Spector ZZ, Menon S, Shwayder M, Bradley DJ, Cohen MI, Sanatani S. Life-threatening event risk in children with Wolff-Parkinson-White Syndrome: a multicenter international study. JACC Clin Electrophysiol. 2018;4(4):433–44.

Atrial Flutter, Typical and Atypical

David T. Huang and Travis Prinzi

Abstract

Atrial flutter is a macroreentrant tachycardia. It is most commonly found in its typical form in which the reentrant circuit travels around the right atrium in a counterclockwise and sometimes clockwise fashion. Atrial flutter can also be a more complex arrhythmia, traveling around scars or other lines of block in either the right or left atrium; these "atypical flutters" are also referred to as macroreentrant non-cavotricuspid isthmus dependent atrial tachycardias.

Mapping and ablation of atrial flutters has become more refined as technology has advanced. Apart from occasional, rare anatomic challenges, typical flutter ablation is fairly straightforward, especially with contact force technology for ablation. While atypical flutter circuits were previously difficult to delineate due to limited point-by-point low-density mapping, new mapping catheters and algorithms have made the discovery and ablation of these circuits more successful in recent years.

D. T. Huang (✉) · T. Prinzi
University of Rochester Medical Center, Rochester, NY, USA
e-mail: David_Huang@URMC.Rochester.edu

© The Author(s), under exclusive license to Springer Nature Switzerland AG 2023
D. T. Huang et al. (eds.), *Cardiac Electrophysiology in Clinical Practice*, In Clinical Practice,
https://doi.org/10.1007/978-3-031-41479-4_7

This chapter will cover the basics of atrial flutter as well as advancements in technology that we now use to treat more complex atypical flutters.

> **Keywords**
>
> Atrial flutter · Typical atrial flutter · Atypical atrial flutter · Macroreentrant tachycardia · Dual loop flutter · Catheter ablation · 3D mapping · Electroanatomic mapping

Incidence and Etiologies

The incidence of atrial flutter is largely unknown due to a lack of organized data in the general population. Most of the epidemiologic data on atrial flutter have been grouped together with data from patients with atrial fibrillation. The estimate for the incidence of new cases of atrial flutter in the United States is around 200,000 per year.

As with atrial fibrillation, atrial flutter occurs more frequently in patients with structural heart disease. Although the causes of atrial flutter are not entirely understood, certain conditions have been implicated or associated with a higher risk for developing atrial flutter. These include hypertension, coronary artery disease, congestive heart failure and valvular heart disease such as those resulting from rheumatic heart disease [1]. It is thought that any condition that leads to an increased stretch and load on the atria can be a potential cause for any atrial arrhythmia. Congenital heart disease, either surgically repaired or not, and cardiac surgery, either involving an incision in the atrium or not, are also common causes of atrial flutter. Other conditions such as an overactive thyroid, fever, lung disease, or even alcohol can be associated with atrial flutter. Many of these mechanisms are still not well delineated, although it appears that inflammation may play a role in the pathogenesis.

Classification

Atrial flutter has been classified several ways. Historically, it has been described as "typical" vs. "atypical," initially based on the rate of the flutter in the atrium and with the most commonly

7 Atrial Flutter, Typical and Atypical

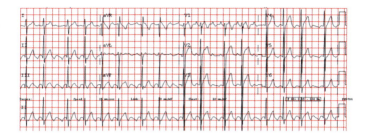

Fig. 7.1 Typical atrial flutter EKG. Notice classic "saw tooth" p waves in inferior leads, and positive p waves in V1 and V2

encountered variant termed as "typical" flutter [2]. In 2001, the North American Society of Pacing and Electrophysiology proposed a different classification system based on mechanism of the flutter as well as the anatomic circuits involved [3]. "Typical" or "Type I" atrial flutter displays a classic pattern of downward deflecting "saw-tooth" flutter waves on the inferior leads of 12 lead EKG and the flutter waves are of a positive polarity (upright) in the early precordial leads, V1 and V2 (see Fig. 7.1). By convention, "Atypical" or "Type II" atrial flutter are those that display any other patterns on the 12 lead EKG.

Mechanisms of Atrial Flutter

Atrial flutter can best be distinguished from atrial tachycardia in that atrial flutter is a reentrant circuit, whereas atrial tachycardia is focal. During atrial flutter, the electrical signal in the atrium traverses around in a fixed circuit. The circuit can involve the entire right or left atrium or just part(s) of the atrium. In contrast, an atrial tachycardia originates from a focal source in the atrium, i.e., a group of cells firing off abnormal electrical activity. Atrial flutter can be distinguished from atrial fibrillation (AF) by the organization of the flutter circuit within the atria. The circuit leading to atrial flutter often is well organized, meaning that the path of the circuit is the same with each flutter cycle length, and it repeats itself over and over again. Occasionally, atrial flutter can involve more than one stable circuit. Atrial flutter is distinguished from

AF in that AF is a much more disorganized atrial arrhythmia. There is no stable circuit in fibrillation. In AF, the signals in the atria are often crashing into themselves or into each other.

In order for a reentering impulse to be continually repetitive as in "Typical" or "Type I" atrial flutter, it needs to be a stable circuit. The stability of the circuit is attributed to the presence of an excitable gap, where the heart tissue trailing the traversing impulse has recovered from refractoriness and is able to be excited again. In addition, there is an area of slow conduction within the circuit. These conditions fulfill the two requirements for impulse reentry (1) different impulse travel speeds or conduction velocities in two pathways where the electrical signals can go through; (2) differential refractoriness of the tissues in these two pathways). The areas of slow conduction can be a result of anatomic variations (variable patterns in cell alignment, the so called "anisotropy", or anatomic structures that are more fibrous and less conducting) or as a result of scar from inflammation, surgery or stretch.

In patients who present with the most commonly encountered atrial flutter ("typical atrial flutter"), this area of slow conduction coincides with the region between the tricuspid valve and the inferior vena cava and bordered by the Eustachian ridge (see Fig. 7.2). This is often referred to as the "cavo-tricuspid isthmus" because it forms a bridge of tissue through which the circuit is sustained. These slow conduction areas often become targets for ablation where if the reentering circuit can be interrupted or cut permanently, then the atrial flutter can be considered cured. This can be achieved with ablation through the circuit resulting in complete conduction block across the isthmus.

The traditional classification of "Atypical" or "Type II" atrial flutter had involved circuits other than the one traveling through the cavo-tricuspid isthmus. With better mapping techniques and improved understanding, these "atypical" atrial flutters have now been defined further. Atypical atrial flutter can involve either the right or the left atrium. It is now well know that ablations in the left atrium, particularly for atrial fibrillation, can result in atrial flutter as an unintended outcome of the ablation procedure. During an ablation for AF, linear ablation lesions create barriers in the left

7 Atrial Flutter, Typical and Atypical

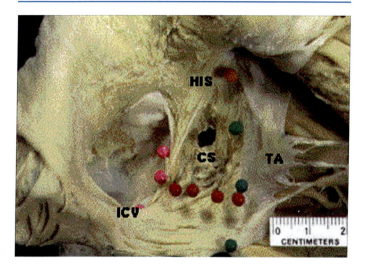

Fig. 7.2 RA anatomy for typical atrial flutter. IVC – Inferior Vena Cava; CS – Coronary Sinus; TA – Tricuspid Annulus; His – Bundle of His

atrium to isolate the areas where fibrillation originates. These barriers, if not contiguous, can have gaps in the line or create areas of slow conduction. This can in turn set up conditions needed for flutter circuits in the left atrium. Some of more commonly encountered circuits, the "roof-dependent" flutters, involve circuits traveling around the right or left pulmonary veins (Fig. 7.4a, b). Another commonly occurring atrial flutter travels around the mitral annulus using the gap between the left inferior pulmonary vein and the mitral annulus (or the so-called left atrial isthmus).

Scarring from inflammation, surgery or ischemia/infarct can also create conditions leading to barriers within the atrial tissue that, in turn, set up the atrium for flutter circuits. Complex circuits have been mapped and reported which lead to another variant of "atypical" atrial flutter. Most atrial flutters involve a single circuit, but there may be multiple circuits involved. One such two-circuit or "dual-loop" example that has been reported involves one circuit that participates in a "typical flutter" fashion, going through the cavo-tricuspid isthmus, and at the same time a secondary cir-

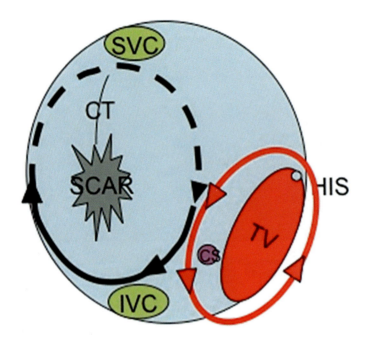

Fig. 7.3 Schematic representation of dual loop atrial flutter

cuit going through a scar area on the more lateral aspect of the right atrium (Fig. 7.3). These circuits traverse through the atrium together in a "figure of 8" pattern, facilitating and sustaining one another (Fig. 7.4a–d). When multiple circuits are involved, there often is a coordinated activation around these circuits, meaning that the signals travel through these circuits at a fixed rate from beat to beat, thus creating a stable flutter. For these more complex flutters, ablation may be needed across multiple circuits in order to terminate the atrial flutter and convert to normal sinus rhythm, as well as to prevent further recurrences of signals traveling around either one of the circuits.

7 Atrial Flutter, Typical and Atypical

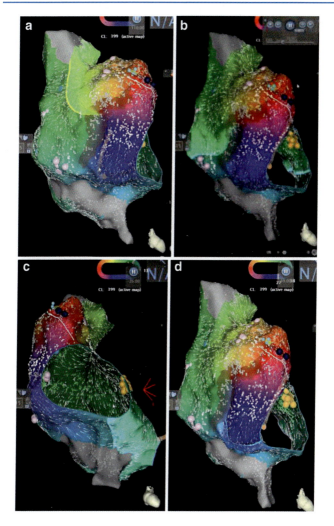

Fig. 7.4 (**a**–**d**) Carto 3 Coherent map of Dual Loop Right Atrial Flutter. The brighter areas of color denote wavefront propagation. In Figure **a**, the wavefront is seen turning around a lateral scar in the RA, with entire TCL around scar. In figure **b**, wavefronts can be seen traversing both lateral and medial walls of RA. In figure **c**, wavefront can be seen using the typical cavotricuspid isthmus. Figure **d** shows the two wavefronts meeting together in a shared common isthmus

Management

Many options are available for the treatment of atrial flutter, and treatment should be tailored to individual patient needs and circumstances. These can range from cautious monitoring to invasive therapy with catheter ablation. As atrial flutter is a non-life-threatening arrhythmic condition, symptomatic control is often the primary goal for therapy. Other important reasons for treating atrial flutter also include reducing the risk of tachycardia-mediated cardiomyopathy and minimizing recurrent heart failure exacerbation.

In general, the goals in managing atrial flutter include: control of ventricular rates during atrial flutter, restoration of regular sinus rhythm, and prevention of thromboembolic events. A wide variety of drugs can be utilized for medical therapy, such as beta blockers or calcium channel blockers that control the ventricular response rate, membrane active antiarrhythmic drugs such as propafenone, flecainide or ibutilide to restore sinus rhythm, and anticoagulants such as warfarin or dabigatran to reduce the risks of embolic events such as stroke.

Catheter based therapy has now become accepted as another first line treatment for patients with atrial flutter, especially ones with "typical" or "type I" variant. It offers a potential curative option and much improved long-term maintenance of sinus rhythm as compared with medical therapy. (ref) The technical aspects of ablation have been discussed in the **Technical Considerations** section of this chapter. The primary aim in ablation for atrial flutter is to interrupt the reentrant circuit permanently. Thus the main strategy in mapping atrial flutter is to locate an isthmus (narrow ridge) of tissue where the electrical impulse in the atrium travels through two electrically inactive boundary areas, such as anatomical structures like the tricuspid valve and the inferior vena cava, or scars. The goal of the ablation needs to be more than the restoration of sinus mechanism. To achieve electrical conduction block across the critical isthmus of the flutter circuit completely is regarded as the successful endpoint. It's important not only that the arrhythmia stop, but that it can never come back.

In patients with atypical flutter that is refractory to conventional curative ablation and medical therapy, ablation of the atrioventricular node is another strategy that can be used to treat patients with atrial flutter. This ablation will induce significant bradycardia, and a pacemaker will be needed to maintain an adequate heart rate. Pacing usually involves single right ventricular lead stimulation. Alternatively, biventricular pacing devices have been used which may improve long term hemodynamic response in patients and lower incidence of heart failure.

Prevention of thromboembolic events with anticoagulation therapy is another main objective in the treatment of patients with atrial flutter. For patients assessed to be at risk, such as those with heart failure, structural heart disease, older age, and prior stroke or transient ischemic attacks, therapy with anticoagulants is recommended. Warfarin has been a mainstay medication traditionally. Newer antithrombin agents such as dabigatran and rivaroxaban have been demonstrated to be effective alternatives.

Technical Considerations

Mapping

The best way to assess atrial flutter and macro-reentrant atrial tachyarrhythmias is by careful and thorough 3-dimensional mapping. The first step is to choose a consistent reference to be "time zero" for the activation map, a fixed location of electrical activation. This needs to be from a catheter that will reliably stay in the same anatomic position recording electrical signals timed consistently with every cycle, so that "time zero" never changes. Usually, the best catheter to use as a reference is a bipolar electrogram (EGM) on the coronary sinus catheter, which should stay in place throughout the entire procedure and sits epicardially to the LA, so is less prone to movement during the manipulation of the mapping catheter. The mapping catheter is manipulated by the operator in the chamber of interest. In atrial flutters, it roves around the atria gathering local electrical activation (EA) data. Prior to recent developments in mapping technology, choosing a reliable reference for timing was often a challenge when CS EGMs were fractionated. New algorithms that analyze all unipolars and bipolars of the CS allow for a stable timing reference in most cases.

Once a reliable reference is chosen, the next step is to set the window of interest (WOI) for activation mapping. Traditionally, local activation time (LAT) mapping for macro-reentrant arrhythmias has been done by calculating 90% of the tachycardia cycle length (TCL), and splitting that number 50/50 on either side of the reference EGM. So if the TCL is 220 ms, the window will be 199 ms, with 98 ms on either side of the reference EGM. So the WOI would be −98 ms to 98 ms. This is a quick method of setting the WOI, and mapping 90% will demonstrate, if the operator is mapping a reentrant circuit and is doing so in the correct chamber, a transition area where the earliest measured signal meets up with the latest measured signal ("early-meets-late"). This helps to confirm that the arrhythmia is indeed originating in the particular chamber mapped, and the details of the impulse circuit demonstrate where the reentrant circuit is traveling.

There are, however, cons to using this method. Because LAT data is collected in reference to an arbitrary "time zero," the "early-meets-late" is also arbitrary. It shows *that* the arrhythmia is reentrant and *where* the circuit is traveling, but it does not serve as a guide for where to ablate. In other words, ablating along the early-meets-late line on the mapping system will not necessarily terminate the arrhythmia. For typical atrial flutter, this hardly matters. In typical atrial flutter, the shortest line between two electrically isolated structures is the cavo-tricuspid isthmus (the ridge of tissue separated by the boundaries of inferior vena cava and the tricuspid valve), and this is what will be regularly targeted for ablation (more on this below).

If, however, the tachycardia is somewhere in the left atrium, or traveling around a scar in either atrium, deciding on a target for curative ablation can be trickier. While the standard 90% TCL, 50/50 window will give the basic data for the reentrant circuit, a more advanced but beneficial algorithm for setting the WOI may be used. Robert DePonti has proposed the following for setting the mapping window: Using this method, the early-meets-late line on the 3D map will be placed in the circuit's mid-diastolic isth-

7 Atrial Flutter, Typical and Atypical

mus (MDI), the zone of slow conduction [4]. In atypical flutters that are less clear, mapping the mid-diastolic isthmus provides a more helpful picture of the tachycardia circuit and may also guide ablation, as the MDI for atypical flutter is usually found in low voltage and scar areas.

$$\text{Backward Interval} = (\text{TCL} - \text{Pwave Duration})/2 \\ + \text{Interval}: \text{PwaveOnset} - \text{REF}$$

$$\text{Forward Interval} = (\text{TCL} - \text{Backward Interval}) \times .9$$

To make it less complicated, the basic concept is to put the P wave in the middle of the window, and to put the "early meets late" portion of the cycle length in the middle of atrial diastole (between two P waves).

The final but crucial step to mapping atrial flutter is correct annotation of the acquired points. This can be challenging when presented with fractionated or double potential EGMs. While mapping algorithms have become better at annotated EGMs, map analysis will always be a crucial part of assessing the accuracy of timing annotation. In the atypical flutter below (dual loop using LA roof and perimitral circuits), the early-meets-late as annotated by the system is unclear. The second image, corrected by a trained mapper and an electrophysiologist evaluating annotation of points in the unclear area, provides a clearer early-meets-late (Fig. 7.5).

Some advanced mapping algorithms have been developed employing some AI to interpret maps when they are unclear. Below is the same map as above with Carto 3's Coherent algorithm applied. The mechanism is quite a bit clearer as far as overall propagation and cleans up all of the false green spaces in the initial map. It does, however, miss the areas of block (white lines) provided by the correctly annotated map.

Finally, some mapping algorithms have been developed that are meant to transcend the tradition difficulties of EA mapping (unstable references, annotation difficulties) by displaying activation data independent of references and the confines of a window of interest. Carto's Ripple Mapping Module, for example, is a propagation algorithm that plays the entirety of each electrogram collected by the high density mapping catheter. Since it

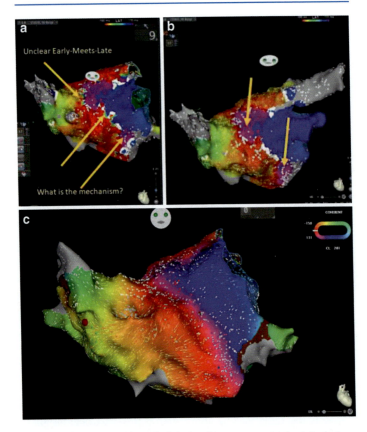

Fig. 7.5 (**a**) has unusual atypical timing that appears non-physiologic (random green areas), where as Figure **b**, edited through careful EGM analysis, has a clear and consistent early-meets-late. (**c**) Carto 3 Coherent Map of the same atypical flutter, which utilizes an algorithm that provides a "best fit" interpretation of the data, cleaning up the unclear early-meets-late area

plays the entire EGM for its duration, it is not limited by having to choose one part of an EGM for timing. Ripple mapping essentially plays the raw EGM data in a propagation video that allows an analysis of electrical wavefronts traversing the chamber.

It is important to remember that all of these algorithms are important voices in the diagnosis of each flutter circuit. While certain mapping tools may appeal more to some than others, using all of them to get a full picture of a complicated circuit is a good idea.

Entrainment

Pacing during any arrhythmia can also aid in the mapping of the electrical circuit. In a reentrant circuit, pacing and the response of the local activation where pacing is taking place can help one locate the critical isthmus of the circuit. The pacing is performed from the selected site at a rate that is slightly faster than the native flutter rate (about 10–15% faster). The pacing site will only capture if pacing is occurring at a faster rate than the native rate. If pacing takes place within an area the circuit traverses through, the first post pacing cycle length ("post pacing interval") should equal to the native flutter cycle length (give or take 10% to permit for conduction delay associated with faster pacing rates and measurement errors). Furthermore, if this is combined with concealed entrainment—if the flutter wave morphology on the surface ECG is identical to the paced p wave or atrial deflection on the surface ECG—then one can be assured that the pacing site is a part of the circuit. This circuit should then be the target of ablation. If the isthmus comprises a small region, a point lesion may suffice in terminating the arrhythmia. On the other hand, if the region is relatively larger in size, as in most flutters, a linear ablation across boundaries of this area, such as the tricuspid valve and the inferior vena cava for "typical" atrial flutter, is needed to terminate the arrhythmia and to prevent any further arrhythmia recurrence through the same circuit and the same isthmus. If the surface ECG atrial waves exhibit a different morphology than during the native flutter, then the pacing is called a manifest or non-concealed entrainment. This site is not part of the circuit and ablation in this area will not be successful in terminating the arrhythmia.

Ablation

The goal of ablation therapy for an arrhythmia involving a reentrant mechanism is to interrupt the circuit permanently so that normal sinus rhythm can be restored and the recurrence of the same arrhythmia can be prevented. Strategies for ablation often target between two electrically inactive structures bordering an area that is critical to the reentrant circuit (called a "critical isthmus" part of the circuit) and to create a line of electrical block in this region. This can cut through the path of the circuit and by taking advantage of the surrounding anatomic structures that do not conduct electrical signals, the barriers to conduction will no longer permit the electrical impulses to reenter leading to a recurrence of the same arrhythmia.

In typical atrial flutter, this ablation is performed at the cavo-tricuspid isthmus (see Fig. 7.2). It is well known that the typical flutter circuit travels through the area between the tricuspid valve and the inferior vena cava. By cutting the conduction through this isthmus region, the electrical impulse cannot travel through this and the surrounding tricupid valve and the inferior vena cava the flutter can be cured. Other areas in the right atrium may potentially be targeted for ablation but these may be impractical because of the larger areas involved and/or proximity to sensitive functional structures such as the sinoatrial or the atrioventricular nodes. The cavo-tricuspid isthmus is readily accessible through an inferior venous approach from the femoral vein and does not contain vital structures to the function of the heart. Therefore, it is an ideal region to target for ablation. In "atypical" atrial flutter, linear lesions are often created between scars, or between a previous ablation line and another electrically isolated structure (e.g., lateral wall right atrial scar to inferior vena cava, or left inferior pulmonary vein isolation line to mitral valve).

Several catheter options and modalities are available for the creation of a linear lesion, including longer-tip radiofrequency ablation catheters (8 or 10 mm), irrigated-tip radiofrequency ablation, or cryoablation. Settings (power-controlled or temperature-controlled) will depend on catheter choice and area being treated.

Where to ablate across the cavo-tricuspid isthmus for typical flutter is an important consideration. The shortest distance across the isthmus is around 6 o'clock on the tricuspid annulus, based on a left anterior oblique projection of the heart. The anatomy there is prone, however, to be associated with diverticulum, or "pouches", in the tissue, making it more difficult to drag an ablation line. A more medial approach (5 o'clock on the same projection) may also have pouches, and it is closer to sensitive structures like the coronary sinus ostium and the atrioventricular node. A lateral approach (7 o'clock) allows you to avoid pouches, but the atrial musculature tends to be thicker and pectinate muscles may also be located here, leading to a lower likelihood of successful transmural ablation lesions. Each patient may have variations on these issues and anatomic along with electrical voltage mapping of the area targeted for ablation can be helpful in selecting the best suitable site for ablation therapy.

When dealing with atypical flutters, determining location for a line of block can be more difficult. In the case of mitral isthmus flutters in the LA, a line is often drawn from a previous left inferior pulmonary vein circumferential isolation line (from an atrial fibrillation ablation) down to the mitral annulus. This area has now been termed as the "left atrial mitral isthmus". Due to the prominence of post-AF ablation atrial flutters observed, electrophysiologists now avoid creating these ablation lines as part of the atrial fibrillation ablation strategy. Nevertheless, these flutters can be observed and is one of the more common atypical atrial flutters that can occur after an atrial fibrillation ablation. Once this type of flutter has been noted to occur spontaneously, the recurrence rate is high and the flutter can often be very persistent leading to more symptoms than the paroxysmal atrial fibrillation. Ablation in the left atrial mitral isthmus region is then needed to eliminate the substrate for this flutter. These ablation lines are notoriously difficult to achieve complete conduction block endocardially within the left atrium and sometimes need to be finished epicardially by ablating within the distal coronary sinus. In the case of LA roof-dependent flutter, linear ablation across roof is created from the right superior pulmonary vein to the left superior pulmonary vein. In the case of scar-mediated atrial flutters, ablation is performed either between two dense scars, or a scar and another electrically isolated structure.

Validation

Successful ablation occurs when bi-directional block is created across a critical isthmus, eliminating the reentering circuit entirely. In typical flutter, this line of block is created between the tricuspid valve and the inferior vena cava. If ablation is performed during atrial flutter, the first step in observing success is the restoration of sinus rhythm. This does not necessarily mean it's time to stop ablating. While the atrial flutter has terminated, one must be certain that no atrial flutter can ever travel through that isthmus again.

There are a few options for confirming bi-directional block across the isthmus. If a Halo catheter has been placed around the tricuspid annulus, or any other kind of 10- or 20-pole catheter has been placed on the lateral wall of the RA, pacing from the coronary sinus will show a proximal-to-distal activation sequence on the Halo (see Fig. 7.6). Pacing in the other direction (from the distal pole of the Halo) will reveal a pattern in which the CS proximal poles will be later than all the poles of the Halo catheter. If,

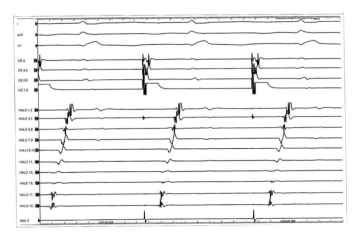

Fig. 7.6 Pacing from CS, Halo activation is proximal to distal. This means the CTI is blocked

7 Atrial Flutter, Typical and Atypical

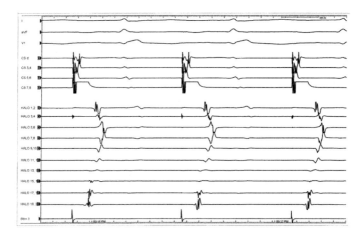

Fig. 7.7 Pacing from CS catheter, activation on Halo is not proximal to distal. This means activation is still passing through the CTI

during CS pacing, there is a curved or "Chevron" activation pattern recorded by the Halo catheter (see Fig. 7.7), CTI block is not complete, and more ablation must be done.

For physicians who do not prefer to have an extra catheter in the heart (Halo or other lateral wall catheter) and would rather use a two-catheter approach (CS catheter and ablation), conduction time can be measured to demonstrate block by placing the ablation catheter on the lateral side of the ablation line. The ablation catheter can be placed on the ablation line to look for double potentials while CS pacing. Double potentials that are separated by at least 90 ms are suggestive of CTI block, and if the interval between double potentials measured consistently ≥90 ms with a maximal variation of 15 ms along the entire ablation line, it can be used to confirm complete block in the cavo-tricuspid isthmus [5].

A 3 dimensional activation map can be used as another method to validate CTI block, and it is also valuable for assessing the breakthrough point, or conduction gap, if block is not complete. Pacing from CS proximal, with the paced catheter as the "time zero" reference (with a window of approximate +20 to +200), an electroanatomic map should show a clear block of conduction along the ablation line. If block is not present, careful and detailed activation mapping along the ablation line should show where electrical activity is still sneaking through the line of block, and this can serve as a guide to finish ablation. The voltage map of the region can be used to observe where tissue along the line is still active with a substantial voltage mapped and serve as another guide to complete the ablation.

Validation can be more complex with atypical flutter ablation lines, but applying the same principle used in the criteria for typical flutter ablation can be adopted to demonstrate bidirectional block across the associated critical isthmus in atypical flutter cases. By placing catheters on either side of the created line of block and pacing in both directions, bidirectional block across the linear lesion can be confirmed with these additional activation maps.

References

1. Granada J, Uribe W, Chyou PH, Maassen K, Vierkant R, Smith PN, Hayes J, Eaker E, Vidaillet H. Incidence and predictors of atrial flutter in the general population. J Am Coll Cardiol. 2000;36(7):2242.
2. Wells JL Jr, MacLean WA, James TN, Waldo AL. Characterization of atrial flutter. Studies in man after open heart surgery using fixed atrial electrodes. Circulation. 1979;60:665.
3. Saoudi N, Cosio F, Waldo A, et al. A classification of atrial flutter and regular atrial tachycardia according to electrophysiological mechanisms and anatomic bases; a Statement from a Joint Expert Group from The Working Group of Arrhythmias of the European Society of Cardiology and the North American Society of Pacing and Electrophysiology. Eur Heart J. 2001;22(14):1162.
4. DePonti R. Treatment of macro-re-entrant atrial tachycardia based on electroanatomic mapping: identification and ablation of the mis-diastolic isthmus. Eur Secur. 2007;9:449–57.
5. Tada H, Oral H, Sticherling C, et al. Double potentials along the ablation line as a guide to radiofrequency line as a guide to radiofrequency ablation of typical atrial flutter. J Am Coll Cardiol. 2001;38(3):750.

A Practical Guide to Catheter Ablation of Atrial Fibrillation

8

Joshua Haswell, Travis Prinzi, and Burr Hall

Abstract

Atrial fibrillation (AF) remains the most common cardiac rhythm disturbance encountered in clinical practice, with rising prevalence over the past 50 years (Lip Gregory et al. Heart 93:542-3, 2007; Kornej et al. Circ Res 127:4-20, 2020; Mou et al. Circ Arrhythm Electrophysiol 11:e006350, 2018). With antiarrhythmic drugs limited by efficacy and side effects, ablation via pulmonary vein isolation (PVI) has become an increasingly common and successful management strategy to control patient symptoms and, in certain populations, lessen morbidity and mortality (Marrouche et al., N Engl J Med 378:417–427, 2018). In this chapter we discuss appropriate patient selection for PVI ablation, the present and upcoming energy modalities used in clinical practice (namely radiofrequency, cryogenic, and pulsed-field), consideration of non-pulmonary vein targets including isolation of the posterior left atrial wall or the vein of Marshall, as well as common procedural complications and strategies to mitigate them including management of periprocedural anticoagulation. We demonstrate a practical step-by-

---

J. Haswell · T. Prinzi · B. Hall (✉)
University of Rochester Medical Center, Rochester, NY, USA
e-mail: Burr_Hall@urmc.Rochester.edu

step guide to AF ablation including anatomical orientation, transseptal puncture, pulmonary vein access, catheter manipulation within the left atrium, and successful ablation guided by intracardiac echocardiography (ICE), fluoroscopy, three-dimensional electro anatomical mapping, and additional industry-specific tools.

Keywords

Atrial fibrillation · Pulmonary vein isolation · Catheter ablation Radiofrequency · Cryoballoon · Intracardiac echo

Introduction

Atrial fibrillation (AF) continues to be the most common cardiac rhythm disturbance encountered in clinical practice. In 2016, The Global Burden of Disease Project estimated a worldwide prevalence of AF around 46.3 million individuals. It is estimated that in the United States alone, there will be between 6 and 16 million individuals with a diagnosis of AF by the year 2050. Based on data from the Framingham Heart Study, the prevalence of AF has increased three-fold over the last 50 years. The lifetime risk estimates for atrial fibrillation are now 1 in 3 for white individuals and 1 in 5 for black individuals [1–3].

Antiarrhythmic drugs can reduce the number of AF episodes and duration, but overall have limited efficacy and are often poorly tolerated by a significant percentage of patients. Pulmonary vein isolation (PVI) is now considered to be a safe and effective therapy in patients with symptomatic atrial fibrillation. The primary goal of AF ablation is to improve patient quality of life by eliminating or significantly reducing the total burden of AF episodes and discontinuing antiarrhythmic drug therapy when possible. AF ablation can also significantly reduce morbidity and mortality in certain patient populations; most notably in patients with heart failure and reduced ejection fraction where AF ablation may be indicated regardless of the presence or absence of symptoms [4].

In this chapter we describe how we have been performing ablation for AF over the past 18 years at the University of Rochester Medical Center. While AF ablation technique may vary across medical institutions, we share our protocol as we have found that the methods that we describe have served us very well from both a safety and efficacy standpoint.

Patient Selection

The primary indication for ablation of AF should be to improve arrhythmia-related symptoms such as palpitations, fatigue, shortness of breath and exercise intolerance. There is little to no data to suggest that AF ablation can reduce mortality in patients without heart failure and reduced ejection fraction, and therefore symptom improvement should be the primary goal of AF ablation. We have seen patients in our practice with asymptomatic AF who are interested in proceeding with AF ablation as an alternative to long-term systemic anticoagulation. The challenge with such an approach is that many patients can have a high prevalence of asymptomatic atrial fibrillation [5]. It has therefore always been our practice not to discontinue systemic anticoagulation post-ablation in patients who have a high risk of stroke as determined by their CHA_2DS_2-VASc score regardless of the patient reported presence or absence of symptoms indicative of recurrent AF. Patients who have a strong desire to discontinue systemic anticoagulation should at the very least undergo longer-term monitoring looking for recurrences of atrial arrhythmias. In our practice, we utilize a combination of 14-day Holter monitors, 30-day mobile cardiac outpatient telemetry monitors, and implantable cardiac monitors that can record continuously for 3 years or more.

Consensus indications for ablation of AF have been well described in the 2019 AHA/ACC/HRS focused update expert consensus statement [6]. While these guidelines are very helpful in determining the appropriateness of AF ablation in a specific patient cohort, it is also imperative that patient preference be carefully considered. AF ablation is a complex procedure with procedural risk, and the risk/benefit ratio of performing such a procedure

Table 8.1 Patient selection for AF ablation

Patient characteristic	Better candidate	Worse candidate
Symptoms	Highly Symptomatic	Asymptomatic
Failed Class I or III antiarrhythmic drugs	>1	0
AF classification	Paroxysmal	Long standing persistent
Age at time of ablation	Younger (<70)	Older (>70)
Left atrial size	<80 cc	>120 cc
Concomitant cardiac disease	No	Yes
Pulmonary disease	No	Yes
Obstructive sleep apnea	No	Yes
Obesity	No	Yes
Prior stroke	No	Yes

must be carefully considered for each patient. There are many clinical and imaging-based variables that can be used to help define the efficacy and procedural risk of AF ablation in an individual patient, which are summarized in Table 8.1.

AF duration is an important predictor of ablation success, with persistent AF being a known independent predictor of AF recurrence post-ablation compared with paroxysmal AF [7], likely due to the progressive nature of AF and associated electrical and structural substrate remodeling in the left atrium. Most trials demonstrating the efficacy of AF ablation were performed in the "paroxysmal" patient population, with the quality and quantity of data concerning outcomes of AF ablation in the non-paroxysmal (i.e. persistent or longstanding persistent) patient population being quite limited. The theory that progressive remodeling of the left atrium in persistent and longstanding persistent AF leads to vulnerable substrate for triggers or re-entry in previously-healthy myocardium has led to multiple attempts to improve the efficacy of persistent AF ablation by targeting additional non-pulmonary vein areas for ablation (e.g. isolated complex fractionated atrial electrograms [CFAEs], linear ablation along the left atrial roof, floor, or mitral isthmus, ethanol-based ablation of the vein of Marshall, etc.). Unfortunately, despite numerous well-designed studies attempting to identify additional ablation targets to consistently improve the efficacy in persistent or longstanding persistent AF, the results have largely been mixed and PVI remains the cornerstone of therapy. A 2014 meta-analysis suggested that PVI combined with linear ablation within the left atrium, but not CFAE ablation, was the most effective strategy [8]. Unfortunately, this was not borne out in the subsequent STAR AF II trial, which randomized patients with persistent AF to PVI, PVI plus CFAE ablation, or PVI plus linear ablation along the left atrial roof and mitral isthmus and found no improvement over PVI alone [9]. Instead, procedural time was significantly shorter with a trend towards increased efficacy in the PVI alone arm. A small randomized clinical trial in 2020 (VENUS) did show some improvement in efficacy by adding ethanol-based ablation of the vein of Marshall to standard radiofrequency ablation (PVI in all patients plus additional targets at operator discretion) [10], but this also added significant procedural time and has not yet been sufficiently validated to become routine practice. At our institution, we typically begin with PVI alone and consider additional ablation targets, including posterior wall isolation with roof and floor lines or less commonly vein of Marshall ablation or mitral lines, for repeat or complex cases.

In our own experience, we have also found that left atrial volume is a major predictor of AF ablation success. In a subset of 88 patients with both paroxysmal and persistent AF at our institution undergoing AF ablation, left atrial volume measured by CT strongly predicted AF recurrence following ablation. The recurrence rate increased from 10% in patients with left atrial volumes of less than 70 cc and increased to over 33% in patients with left atrial volumes between 110 and 129 cc. In patients with a left atrial volume of 130 cc or larger the recurrence rate after ablation was more than 90% and appeared to function as a threshold for failure [11] (Fig. 8.1).

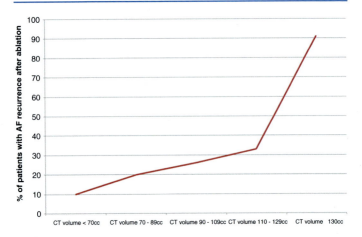

Fig. 8.1 Failure rate after AF ablation depending on left atrial volume by CT. As shown in the ROC analysis, the frequency of AF recurrence after ablation increases as left atrial volume increases. The recurrence rate increase from 10% in patients with small atria with volumes <70 cc and increases to over 33% in patients with left atrial volumes between 110–129 cc. A left atrial volume of at least 130 cc, as measured by CT, appears to function as a threshold. Failure rate in patients with a volume of 130 cc or larger had an AF recurrence rate of more than 90%

Modalities of Atrial fibrillation Ablation

The most commonly used energy sources for isolation of the pulmonary veins are point-by-point radiofrequency (RF) current, which leads to cellular necrosis by tissue heating, and circumferential cryogenic energy delivered by balloon-based systems to cause cellular necrosis by tissue freezing. RF ablation commonly utilizes electro-anatomical mapping systems to decrease the overall fluoroscopic time as well as provide additional data on the underlying left atrial substrate, and offers the flexibility of easily targeting non-pulmonary vein AF triggers or concurrent arrhythmias (e.g. atrial flutter) at the time of PVI. Cryoablation offers a faster procedural time with a shorter learning curve, but is unable to target non-pulmonary vein triggers and can be associated with higher radiation exposure due to commonly-utilized pulmonary vein angiography to confirm adequate occlusion by the balloon prior to delivery of cryogenic energy. There are also instances where patients may have challenging pulmonary vein anatomy on pre-procedural imaging such as very superior pulmonary vein ostium or common ostium that may be better treated with radiofrequency ablation. In the case of common ostium, cryoballoon ablation can still be very effective but may require segmental freeze lesions on both the superior and inferior aspects of the common ostium.

Overall safety and efficacy data suggest these two modalities are similar, with one 2016 randomized trial showing 65% of patients with symptomatic, drug-refractory paroxysmal AF remained free from clinical recurrence over a 1.5 year mean follow-up [12], and another 2019 study identifying a one-year freedom-from-recurrence rate of 53% [13]. Both studies showed no significant difference with regard to overall safety outcomes. The lower success rate seen in the latter study was likely driven by subclinical or asymptomatic AF identified by implantable loop recorder monitoring, which was employed universally in that study while the former used periodic electrocardiograms and Holter monitors to monitor for recurrence. This also highlights one of the common pitfalls encountered when assessing ablation success, as the more modest 53% freedom-from-first-recurrence rate seen in that study can easily obfuscate the more clinically relevant decrease in overall AF burden that can be seen following AF ablation (99% in that case).

Pulsed-field ablation (PFA) is a promising new ablation modality that may be the next major advance in the field. Unlike RF or cryoablation, which achieve cell death by delivery of thermal energy, PFA is a non-thermal modality that uses high amplitude pulsed electrical fields to ablate tissue via irreversible electroporation. In this process, the application of a local electrical field leads to increased plasma cell membrane permeability and eventual cell death via induced apoptosis. It has the potential to be delivered almost instantaneously, taking effect within a single heartbeat instead of requiring seconds-to-minutes of prolonged contact for delivery of thermal energy. Cardiomyocytes appear to be particularly susceptible to irreversible electroporation, whereas nearby tissues of concern including the esophagus, phrenic nerves, pulmonary veins, and coronary arteries are relatively resistant to injury [14]. This, combined with the cellular specificity and sparing of the extracellular matrix, has the potential to offer a faster and safer ablation technology. Initial studies have indeed been promising with favorable durability and safety outcomes [15], but this data remains isolated to nonrandomized trials without adequate comparator groups at this time and larger multicenter, randomized trials are needed before this can be adopted into routine clinical practice.

Complications of Atrial fibrillation Ablation

Over the past decade, there have been significant improvements in catheter ablation techniques. Widespread use of intracardiac echocardiography (ICE), 3-dimensional mapping, steerable sheaths, contact force catheters and balloon-based technologies have all played a role in reducing complications. Pericardial effusion, stroke, and atrioesophageal fistula formation remain the most serious complications related to AF ablation. The National inpatient sample database showed a reduction in complication and mortality rates from 2011 through 2014 as compared to the time period from 2000 through 2010. However, this same database again reported higher complication rates from 2011 through 2014. This likely reflects a larger number of newer and inexperienced operators performing AF ablation and it is well known that complication rates are significantly higher in lower volume, less experienced centers [16, 17]. It is encouraging, however, that serious complications are rare in high-volume centers with extensive operator experience over time. In an individual high-volume tertiary care referral center, serious complications related to ablation of atrial fibrillation were < 1% with zero deaths in over 10,000 patients undergoing ablation for atrial fibrillation. There were no atrioesophogeal fistulas seen in the entire cohort of over 10,000 patients [18].

Complications associated with AF ablation may be related in part to regional differences in left atrial transmural wall thickness. To investigate this, we measured transmural left atrial wall thickness in 34 human heart specimens using calipers in five anatomic areas frequently targeted during AF ablation (anterior wall, septum, mitral isthmus, posterior wall, and roof). The roof was the thinnest region measuring significantly less than each other area. The septum was the thickest area [19]. Significant regional differences exist among the different anatomic areas within the left atrium and lower power and temperature should be used in anatomic regions known to have thinner transmural wall thickness.

Patients undergoing catheter ablation of atrial fibrillation are at increased risk of thromboembolic events during, immediately following, and for several days-to-months after their ablation [20]. The prothrombotic state associated with damaged left atrial endothelium will result in transiently elevated risk of thromboembolism, even in patients previously identified as low-risk for such events prior to catheter ablation. Anticoagulation can effectively diminish these risks but carries a prerequisite risk of increased periprocedural bleeding including access-site complication, cardiac tamponade, or hemothorax. This can make periprocedural anticoagulant management quite challenging. Patients with a CHA_2DS_2-VASc score of at least 2 are generally started on therapeutic anticoagulation at least 3 weeks prior to ablation. The use of warfarin to target an INR 2.0–3.0 was historically a common strategy for this but is increasingly uncommon at present, particularly after the 2019 AHA/ACC/HRS focused update on management of patients with atrial fibrillation specifically recommended the use of a non-vitamin K oral anticoagulant (NOAC) over warfarin in NOAC-eligible patients with AF (Class IA) [6]. When warfarin is still utilized, periprocedural continuation without interruption or bridging, provided the INR is within therapeutic range, has become the most accepted practice. This, in part, follows from a large randomized 2014 trial that randomized patients to uninterrupted warfarin therapy vs discontinuation 2–3 days pre-ablation with enoxaparin bridging and demonstrated a significantly higher risk of stroke or TIA in the bridged group compared to the uninterrupted group (4.9% vs 0.25%) [21]. This same study demonstrated no significant difference in the rate of major bleeding events, with minor bleeding events also favoring the uninterrupted strategy (22% vs 4.1%).

NOAC agents (e.g. apixaban, dabigatran, edoxaban, and rivaroxaban) have a more rapid onset of action, shorter half-life, and more predictable dose response compared to warfarin. A growing amount of evidence has suggested similar or improved efficacy for peri-ablation anticoagulation, as compared with warfarin, which led to the 2017 HRS/EHRA/ECAS/APHRS/SOLAECE expert consensus statement on catheter and surgical ablation of AF recommending continuation of dabigatran or rivaroxaban peri-ablation without interruption (Class I) [20]. Due to limited evidence at the time, the remaining NOAC agents (apixaban, edoxaban) were given Class IIa recommendations for uninterrupted continuation, and it was also acknowledged that holding 1–2 doses of any NOAC prior to AF ablation is reasonable (Class IIa). These guidelines were based on the results of the RE-CIRCUIT study, demonstrating improved safety with uninterrupted dabigatran vs uninterrupted warfarin (major bleeding during and up to 8 weeks postablation 1.6% vs 6.9%) [22], and Venture-AF, a smaller study comparing interrupted rivaroxaban vs uninterrupted warfarin with no major bleeding or cardioembolic events seen in the rivaroxaban arm [23]. Since publication of those guidelines, the AXAFA–AFNET 5 and ELIMINATE-AF trials have demonstrated non-inferiority of uninterrupted apixaban and edoxaban, respectively, vs uninterrupted warfarin for catheter ablation of AF [24, 25]. Our practice is generally to hold 1–2 doses of a NOAC pre-ablation depending on a patient's individual risk profile with prompt post-procedural resumption, or continue warfarin uninterrupted.

Approach to the Left Atrium

Trans-septal puncture (TSP) is the conventional approach to accessing the left atrium. TSP can be challenging even for experienced physicians. In our laboratory, we rely heavily on intracardiac echo (ICE) to perform TSP in a safe and efficient manner.

8 A Practical Guide to Catheter Ablation of Atrial Fibrillation

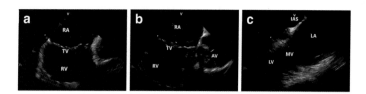

Fig. 8.2 Visualizing the interatrial septum on ICE. (**a**) The ICE Home View clearly visualizes the right atrium (RA), tricuspid valve (TV) and right ventricle (RV). (**b**) Slight posterior rotation of the ICE catheter from the home position bring the aortic valve into view. (**c**) Continued posterior rotation of the ICE catheter from the aortic valve view now brings the interatrial septum (IAS), left atrium (LA), mitral valve (MV), and left ventricle (LV) into view

The ICE catheter is initially advanced into the mid right atrium (RA) in a neutral position. The initial goal is to find the home view which visualizes the RA, tricuspid valve (TV) and right ventricle (RV) (Fig. 8.2a). From the home view, slight clockwise posterior rotation is applied to the catheter until the aortic valve is clearly visualized (Fig. 8.2b). Additional posterior rotation of the ICE catheter will bring the interatrial septum (IAS), left atrium (LA), mitral valve (MV) and left ventricle (LV) into view (Fig. 8.2c).

Further posterior rotation of the ICE catheter will bring into view the left atrial appendage (LAA) (Fig. 8.3a). The ideal site for trans-septal puncture is within an ICE image that is slightly posterior to the LAA view but not so posterior that the pulmonary veins (PVs) are viewed completely. While a more posterior TSP with the PVs clearly in view on ICE will provide for a straightforward and coaxial approach to the left superior and left inferior pulmonary veins (LSPV, LIPV), it will be more challenging to approach the right superior and inferior veins (RSPV, RIPV). This is especially true in a patient with a smaller left atrium where there is very little space between the site of the TSP and the anterior ostium of the RIPV, in which case a slightly more anterior TSP location is helpful. After visualizing the LAA on ICE, the catheter is again rotated slightly posteriorly until the left pulmonary veins come into view (Fig. 8.3b, c). It is important to understand that the ostium of the LIPV is posterior to that of the

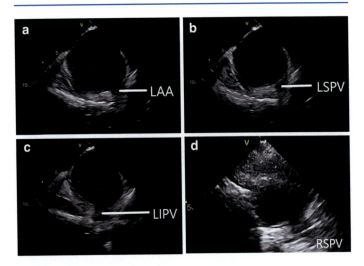

Fig. 8.3 Identification of left atrial anatomy. Intracardiac echo view of the interatrial septum and left atrial appendage (LAA) (**a**), left superior pulmonary vein (LSPV) (**b**), left inferior pulmonary vein (LIPV) (**c**), and right superior pulmonary vein (RSPV) (**d**)

LSPV. Therefore, it is often not possible to view both the LSPV and LIPV in the same ICE projection and more posterior rotation of the catheter is required to clearly visualize the LIPV. After clearly viewing the left sided pulmonary veins, the ICE catheter is advanced superiorly and then additional clockwise posterior rotation is applied to view the right sided pulmonary veins (Fig. 8.3d).

We utilize an 8.5 French Swartz sheath with introducer (Abbott medical) for the TSP. Initially the guide wire is advanced into the left subclavian vein and the sheath and introducer is advanced to the level of the left brachiocephalic vein. The initial orientation of the sheath within the left brachiocephalic vein allows the introducer to fall directly on the fossa ovalis when pulling inferiorly without the need for significant anterior or posterior rotation. Once the sheath and introducer are in place, the transseptal needle is advanced while flushing with heparin saline until the tip of the needle is just proximal to the distal end of the introducer as visualized on Fluoroscopy. We choose to use a radiofrequency trans-

8 A Practical Guide to Catheter Ablation of Atrial Fibrillation

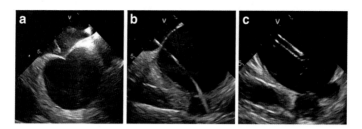

Fig. 8.4 Transseptal puncture and left atrial access. (**a**) ICE image showing clear tenting of the introducer on the fossa ovalis immediately prior to transseptal puncture. (**b**) Guide wire advanced into the LSPV prior to advancing the sheath across the fossa ovalis. (**c**) Confirmation of sheath in the LA. LSPV and LIPV are also visualized

septal needle (Baylis Medical) to facilitate TSP. The sheath and transseptal needle are then pulled down in unison in an inferior direction until clear tenting is visualized on the fossa ovalis with the ICE catheter (Fig. 8.4a). It is important that the hub of the sheath and transseptal needle are coaxial and typically positioned in the 4:30 position as they are pulled down to the fossa ovalis. After clear tenting is visualized on the ICE image with the introducer, the transseptal needle is advanced just distally to the tip of the introducer and radiofrequency energy is applied to cross the interatrial septum. We always attach the transseptal needle to a manifold so that either saline or contrast can be injected immediately following TSP to confirm that bubbles/contrast are visualized in the main chamber of the left atrium (LA) on ICE. Following this confirmation, the transseptal needle is removed and a guide wire is advanced through the introducer into the LSPV (Fig. 8.4b). We do not advance the sheath into the LA until the guide wire is visualized on ICE to be within the LSPV. This ensures that the sheath/introducer will not fall into the LA appendage or other structures when force is applied to cross the interatrial septum. Finally, sheath placement within the LA is confirmed on ICE images (Fig. 8.4c). Heparin is given either immediately prior to TSP or immediately after. We maintain an ACT between 350–400 during AF ablation procedures.

Catheter Manipulation and Radiofrequency Ablation within the Left Atrium and Pulmonary Veins

Once access to the left atrium has been achieved, it is important to understand the anatomic location of the pulmonary vein ostium/orientation, the left atrial appendage, and mitral annulus both on fluoroscopy and three dimensional electroanatomic maps (Fig. 8.5). While we predominantly rely on three-dimensional electro anatomical mapping, it is still very useful to have a clear understanding of the fluoroscopic location of the pulmonary vein ostia and the relationship of the ostia to the cardiac border and spine, which varies significantly between individual patients. This serves to increase the safety of the procedure with fluoroscopic confirmation that the ablation catheter is well outside the pulmonary vein ostia.

Catheter manipulation within the left atrium can be broken down into the pulmonary veins and six major anatomic regions: right anterior wall, right inferior wall, left anterior/ridge, left posterior wall, left atrial roof, and appendage. If one were to draw an imaginary line down the middle of the left atrium, it is our preference to use AP or shallow RAO fluoroscopic views when manipu-

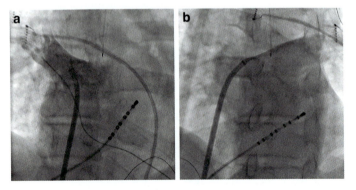

Fig. 8.5 Fluoroscopic location of the right (**a**) and left (**b**) superior pulmonary veins. Esophageal temperature probe is also visualized

lating the ablation catheter to the right of that line and LAO for any catheter movement to the left of that line.

The pulmonary vein ostium are posterior structures within the left atrium. As such, posterior clockwise torque on the catheter and sheath is necessary to access the veins. The left superior pulmonary vein (LSPV) can be entered by directly advancing the ablation catheter from the trans-septal site while clocking the catheter and sheath in a posterior direction. It can be virtually impossible to define the left atrial appendage from the LSPV on two-dimensional fluoroscopy. It is therefore imperative that one carefully looks at the local atrial electrogram as the catheter is being advanced into the LSPV. If the catheter is advanced in too much of an anterior direction, the left atrial appendage can be entered inadvertently and this would be associated with a large amplitude atrial electrogram which should immediately be recognized by the operator. This is in contrast to what one would expect when advancing the catheter into the LSPV which reveals a diminishing amplitude of the atrial electrogram. The left inferior pulmonary vein can be entered by maintaining the same posterior torque and advancing the catheter slightly in the inferior direction. The real time impedance should also be carefully monitored. A high impedance (over 110 ohms) would suggest that the catheter is too distal within the pulmonary vein and ablation should then be avoided.

The right superior pulmonary vein (RSPV) is easily accessed by pulling the catheter out of the LSPV and clocking the sheath and catheter across the high posterior wall until the catheter falls into the RSPV. After mapping the RSPV the catheter can be rotated in a further clockwise direction until it falls out of the vein onto the high anterior wall of the left atrium. At this point the sheath and the catheter can be pulled down together in an inferior direction to the level of the trans-septal puncture to obtain the remainder of the anteroseptal wall (Fig. 8.6).

The right inferior pulmonary vein (RIPV) and surrounding left atrium can be one of the most difficult anatomic regions of the left atrium to reach. This is especially true in patients with smaller left atrial volumes where there is very little distance between the trans-septal puncture site and the ostium of the RIPV. The ostium

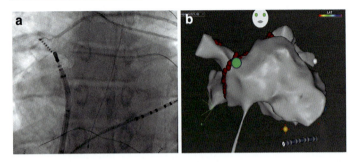

Fig. 8.6 Approach to the anterior wall outside of the RSPV. Corresponding AP fluoroscopic image (**a**) and location (green circle) on three-dimensional electro anatomical map (**b**). Clockwise anterior torque of the ablation catheter from an initial location within the right superior pulmonary vein will result in the catheter falling on the right anterior left atrial wall

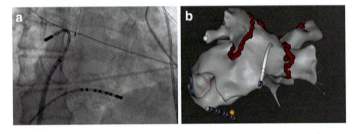

Fig. 8.7 Approach to the right posterior wall and right inferior pulmonary vein. Catheter position shown on corresponding AP fluoroscopy (**a**) and three-dimensional electro-anatomical map (**b**) views. The sheath is directed toward the left. The ablation catheter is then positioned in the opposite direction of the sheath and moved in an inferior and superior direction to approach the entire right posterior wall

of the RIPV is located much more posteriorly than any of the other veins which adds to the challenge of entering this vein and performing ablation around its' entire circumference. When accessing the RIPV, it is our preference to point the sheath toward the LSPV. The catheter is then deflected more than 180 degrees with posterior (counter clockwise) torque until the RIPV is entered (Fig. 8.7). The catheter will not leave the fluoroscopic cardiac silhouette as it does with the other three veins because of the very posterior direction of the RIPV. The right posterior wall and low right anterior wall below the trans-septal puncture site can then be mapped from this configuration by counter clockwise or clockwise catheter rotation respectively.

There are two equally effective methods to both map and ablate along the left atrial roof. The roof of the left atrium is not a flat structure. The roof immediately outside of the LSPV is much more superior than the roof anatomy as it enters the RSPV. This superior to inferior direction of the roof must be taken into account as the catheter is manipulated across the left atrial roof. In an AP fluoroscopic view, the tip of the ablation catheter can be placed in the ostium of the RSPV with the sheath pointed toward the left. The curvature of the catheter is then relaxed allowing the catheter to fall across the roof from right to left (Fig. 8.8). Alternatively, the catheter can be placed into the ostium of the LSPV. The catheter and sheath are then clocked together in a sequential fashion across the posterior aspect of the roof until the ostium of the RSPV is reached. With this method local esophageal temperature must be carefully monitored given the more posterior roof line that is created.

The ridge of the left atrium is located between the anterior ostium of the LSPV and the left atrial appendage. There is sig-

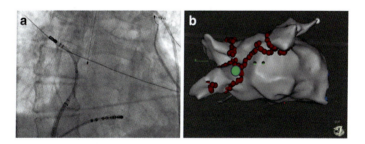

Fig. 8.8 Approach to the left atrial roof. Corresponding catheter position in AP fluoroscopic (**a**) and three-dimensional electro anatomical map (green circle) (**b**) views. To ablate along the left atrial roof, the sheath is pointed to the left and the ablation catheter is positioned in the opposite direction with the distal tip just outside of the RSPV. From this position, the ablation catheter curve is slowly released, thus allowing the catheter to sweep the roof ending at the ostium of the LSPV

nificant anatomic variation to this structure between patients. Higher power settings are often required to achieve bidirectional electrical block along the ridge. The ridge can be ablated from the pulmonary venous or appendage side. It is our preference to ablate along the venous side of the ridge. The ablation catheter is advanced into the LSPV and the sheath is advanced well into the left atrium over the catheter. The catheter is then withdrawn as counterclockwise torque is applied to the sheath. Ablation is performed when both an acceptable electrogram and impedance is obtained. This is one area of the left atrium where more sheath support is required. Without the sheath support, small anterior or posterior movements of the catheter will cause it to fall into the left atrial appendage or LSPV respectively (Fig. 8.9).

The left atrial appendage is usually easily mapped. It is one of the most anterior structures within the left atrium. Advancing the catheter from the trans-septal site toward the LSPV with substantially more anterior torque will allow the catheter to fall into the appendage. It is important to predominately map the base of the appendage because advancing the catheter too far into the appendage can dramatically increase the risk of perforation and is unnecessary for the ablation of AF. In some patients the left atrial appendage can protrude anteriorly over the mitral annulus rather

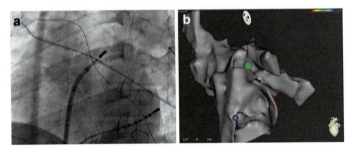

Fig. 8.9 Catheter manipulation at the left atrial ridge between the LSPV and appendage. Corresponding fluoroscopic view (**a**) and three-dimensional electro anatomical map (green circle) (**b**). The ablation catheter is advanced into the LSPV. Counter clockwise torque is then applied to the sheath and catheter as the catheter is pulled back into the sheath until it lands on the ridge. Further counterclockwise rotation will cause the catheter to fall into the appendage

8 A Practical Guide to Catheter Ablation of Atrial Fibrillation

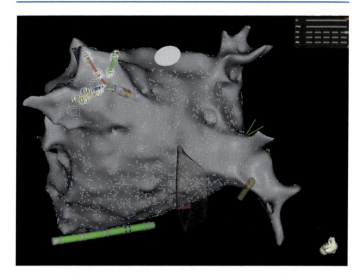

Fig. 8.10 High density mapping catheter utilized for anatomical mapping. Position of catheter in the LSPV

than in the more common anterior superior direction. This anatomic variation should be recognized if no clear left atrial appendage is seen in the usual anatomic location.

While the entire left atrium can be mapped with the ablation catheter alone, it is both more efficient and anatomically accurate to utilize a multipole high density mapping catheter. These high-density catheters are designed to create high density precise anatomical maps with minimal catheter manipulation (Fig. 8.10). These catheters can simultaneously obtain anatomic, voltage and activation mapping points. The approach to the designated anatomic regions of the left atrium as described above are identical for both the ablation and high-density mapping catheters.

Obtaining activation and voltage maps of the left atrium with high-density mapping catheters during coronary sinus pacing can be especially useful in patients presenting for repeat ablation procedures. Areas of higher voltage and conduction into the pulmonary veins which represent sites of pulmonary vein electrical reconnection can easily be identified and then ablated. In addition

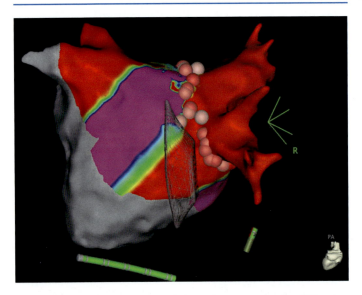

Fig. 8.11 Post pulmonary vein isolation voltage map showing diffuse low voltage/scar medial to the ablation lines

to coronary sinus and pulmonary vein pacing to prove entrance and exit block, we also routinely obtain post-ablation voltage maps as another measure of proving isolation (Fig. 8.11).

Over the last several years, we have exclusively utilized contact force ablation catheters for radiofrequency PVI. Contact force catheters ensure that enough tissue contact is achieved for adequate lesion formation while avoiding excessive contact which may result in tissue injury. There is no consensus on the ideal amount of contact force and electrophysiology labs differ in their goal contact force ranges. We prefer a tissue contact force of between 8–20 g within the left atrium.

In addition to contact force catheters, we have found that using ablation index (Biosense Webster, Inc., Diamond Bar, CA) allows us to achieve PVI more efficiently leading to a reduction in overall procedure times. Ablation index incorporates power, contact force and time in an effort to estimate ablation lesion depth. Utilizing ablation index has been shown to result in a high level of durable PVI with good clinical success [26]. Previous studies have suggested ablation tag index target values as 550 for the anterior wall and 380 for the posterior wall to prevent both acute and delayed pulmonary vein reconnection [27, 28].

Lastly, we have also found that bi-directional guiding sheaths have proven to be very useful for achieving PVI. The bi-directional guiding sheaths provide for enhanced stability and accurate positioning of the ablation catheter as compared to performing the ablation with a standard non-directional sheath. Some of the bi-directional sheaths also allow for sheath visualization on the three-dimensional electroanatomic map which can help to substantially reduce fluoroscopy exposure both to the patient and operator. When using a bi-directional sheath, the ablation catheter is advanced just distally to the tip of the sheath and essentially all of the manipulation during ablation is performed by moving the bi-directional sheath inferiorly or superiorly with the ablation catheter in a fixed position (Fig. 8.12).

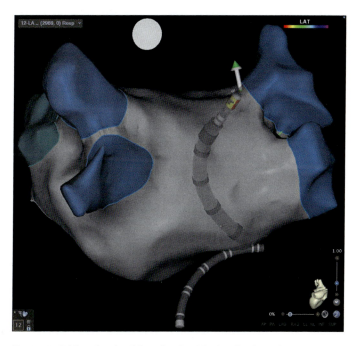

Fig. 8.12 Bidirectional guiding sheath with visualization of the sheath on three-dimensional electro anatomical map. The ablation catheter is positioned just distal to the tip of the sheath and all manipulation is performed with the bi-directional sheath itself

Cryoballoon Ablation

Cryoballoon ablation can serve as a very effective and efficient means to achieve pulmonary vein isolation in most patients with similar efficacy to that of radiofrequency ablation. The operator must be aware of and monitor balloon-tissue contact, time to pulmonary vein isolation, and maximal nadir temperatures. As with any current ablation modality, the risk for damage to collateral tissue exists and esophageal temperature as well as phrenic nerve conduction must be carefully monitored during the freezing application.

We routinely utilize the larger 28-mm balloon (Arctic Front Advance, Medtronic Inc., Minneapolis, MN) to ensure a wider and more proximal ablation lesion. We typically approach the left sided veins first. This allows more time for any paralytic agents that may have been used during anesthesia induction to dissipate prior to attempted pacing of the phrenic nerve during cryoballoon ablation of the right sided pulmonary veins. The Achieve mapping catheter (Medtronic Inc., Minneapolis, MN) is advanced into the LSPV. The Achieve mapping catheter should be placed as proximal as possible while still allowing it to act as a guide for stability of the balloon. Placing the Achieve mapping catheter too distally within the pulmonary vein will make it impossible to view pulmonary vein potentials and evaluate time to isolation during the freezing application. The balloon is then advanced while holding the Achieve catheter in a stable position until the balloon tip is at the ostium of the vein. At this point, the balloon is inflated. The balloon should appear as a round ball on fluoroscopy. A narrowing (goose beak appearance) of the distal balloon suggest that the balloon is positioned too far into the pulmonary vein and should be pulled back. After balloon inflation, the sheath is advanced to the surface of the balloon and gentle pressure is applied to the sheath as the distal tip of the balloon is pushed to the ostium of the vein. With the balloon in position, we then inject contrast through a manifold to evaluate for retention of contrast within the pulmonary vein which indicates balloon/pulmonary vein occlusion (Fig. 8.13). In addition to evaluating pulmonary vein occlusion

8 A Practical Guide to Catheter Ablation of Atrial Fibrillation

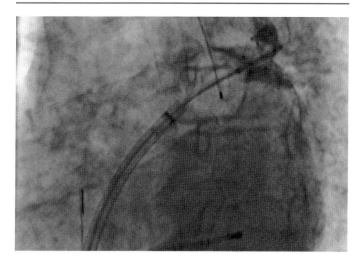

Fig. 8.13 Contrast injection with retention indicating excellent balloon occlusion of the LSPV. Also noted is the esophageal temperature probe which is placed directly posterior to the balloon

with the use of contrast injection, we also routinely utilize doppler on intra-cardiac echo. Doppler can be very useful for patients with a contrast allergy and also can lead to reduction in fluoroscopy usage (Fig. 8.14).

The duration of the freeze is typically between 180 and 240 seconds. During the first minute of the freeze, we like to see a temperature of −30°C by 30 s and −40°C by 60 s. If we are not achieving these temperatures, more forward pressure is applied to the sheath until the goal temperature/time curve is achieved. Alternatively, if temperature is dropping too rapidly, all forward pressure is released. The amount of forward pressure applied or released during the first 60 seconds of the freeze is critical to being able to continue with the freeze for the entire desired time duration. Multiple studies have described the importance of time to pulmonary vein isolation associated with cryoballoon ablation [29–31]. In accordance with these prior studies, we like to achieve PVI with a time to isolation of 60 s or less which has been associated with durable PVI. When clear evidence of PVI occurs by

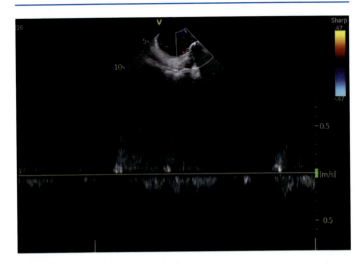

Fig. 8.14 Intra-cardiac echo image showing doppler applied at the contact point of the cryoballoon and pulmonary vein. The doppler pattern shows complete occlusion of the pulmonary vein with the balloon

60 s, we will not extend the freezing lesion time duration beyond 180 s. However, if PVI is not achieved by 60 s or clear pulmonary vein potentials cannot be visualized, we will use a freezing duration of 240 s assuming that phrenic nerve conduction is adequate and esophageal intra-luminal temperatures are stable.

It is critical to monitor intra-luminal esophageal temperatures and phrenic nerve conduction during cryoballoon ablation. We adjust the esophageal temperature probe before every freeze to ensure that it is directly in line with the cryoballoon (Fig. 8.13). Previous studies have recommended a minimal esophageal temperature of >10–15 °C to minimize the chance of esophageal tissue injury [32–35]. We are typically more conservative and will discontinue cryoballoon ablation for luminal esophageal temperatures of less than 30 °C.

Injury to the phrenic nerve can occur when applying cryoballoon ablation to the RSPV and RIPV based on the close anatomic relationship of the phrenic nerve and right sided pulmonary veins. We monitor phrenic nerve conduction by directly capturing and

8 A Practical Guide to Catheter Ablation of Atrial Fibrillation

pacing the phrenic nerve. This is achieved by utilizing a decapolar catheter inserted into the right subclavian/axillary vein and pacing between electrodes one and ten (Fig. 8.15). During the cryoballoon ablation, we start pacing at 20 s into the freeze as to not abruptly dislodge the balloon at the onset of pacing. We then manually feel for diaphragmatic capture and come off ablation for any reduced response. It is critical that the position of all of the electrodes on the pacing catheter are superior to the level of the cryoballoon. Placing the pacing electrodes inferiorly to the level of the cryoballoon can result in phrenic nerve injury that would not be detected while manually palpating for diaphragmatic capture.

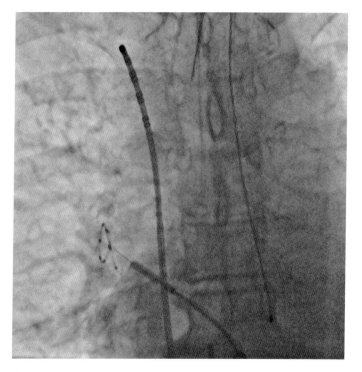

Fig. 8.15 Decapolar pacing catheter placed in right axillary vein for phrenic nerve capture. All electrodes are placed superior to the level of the cryoballoon

Remote Magnetic Navigation-Guided Pulmonary Vein Isolation

Remote magnetic navigation (RMN) catheter ablation has been shown to be a feasible and safe technique to achieve PVI with long-term effectiveness [36, 37]. Potential advantages of RMN catheter ablation are catheter contact and stability as well as the potential for reduced risk of complications secondary to the atraumatic design of the RMN ablation catheter. We have previously described our own experience with RMN for the ablation of AF in 30 consecutive patients [38]. Seventy seven percent of this small patient cohort had persistent atrial fibrillation with an average left atrial volume of 95.4 ± 33.2 ml. These patients were compared to 61 patients undergoing AF ablation with a standard PVI ablation procedure. The rates of final PVI for the individual pulmonary veins for RMN and standard PVI approaches were similar (86.7% versus 89.8% respectively, $p = 0.67$ (Fig. 8.16). However, we did

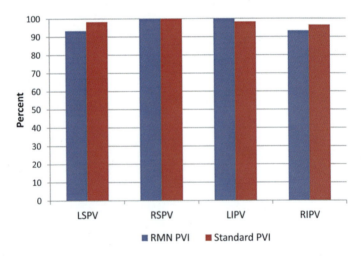

Fig. 8.16 Final individual pulmonary vein isolation rates for remote magnetic navigation and standard ablation techniques. LSPV: left superior pulmonary vein; LIPV: left inferior pulmonary vein; RSPV: right superior pulmonary vein; RIPV: right inferior pulmonary vein

find that anatomic ablation alone with RMN catheter ablation was insufficient to achieve acceptable rates of PVI. In other words, even though RMN catheter ablation may offer improved catheter stability and endocardial contact during radiofrequency application, it is still necessary to utilize an electrogram based approach with a circumferential 20 pole catheter (Lasso) within the pulmonary vein ostium to insure high rates of electrical isolation. No significant procedural complications were noted with either the standard or RMN-guided PVI.

Conclusions

Ablation has become a commonly-used and effective means of suppressing AF burden, both for symptom control and, in some cases, a morbidity and mortality benefit [4]. As the global burden of AF continues increasing, we suspect that ablation will become an increasingly common treatment strategy. Careful patient selection favoring individuals who are younger, healthier, symptomatic, and paroxysmal with smaller left atrial volumes can improve the likelihood of procedural success [11]. At present, PVI remains the most standard approach to AF ablation, either by RF or cryogenic energy, with additional ablation targets (e.g. posterior wall isolation, vein of Marshall ethanol ablation) sometimes considered for complex, persistent, or recurrent cases [8–10]. Pulsed-field ablation is a promising new frontier that may offer a faster and/or safer non-thermal energy modality in the upcoming years [14, 15]. Periprocedural anticoagulation can generally be safely managed with minimal or no interruption to patients' warfarin or NOAC regimens [20–25]. Transseptal left atrial access can be safely performed with ICE guidance, which can also be quite useful for identification of cardiac anatomy including the pulmonary veins and left atrial appendage. Intraprocedural catheter manipulation can be guided by fluoroscopy or three-dimensional electro anatomical mapping software, with both often utilized in many of our cases. High density mapping catheters are a more accurate and efficient means of creating precise anatomical maps with minimal catheter manipulation. Serious complications are rare, particularly at high-volume centers with extensive operator experience, but it remains important to monitor safety parameters such as esophageal temperature and phrenic nerve conductance during the procedure. Activation and voltage mapping are useful adjuvants, particularly in repeat ablations, and additional tools including contact force catheters, ablation indices, and bi-directional guiding sheaths have all helped to improve our efficiency and procedural success. With appropriate patient selection, operator expertise, and modern technology AF ablation can be a safe, effective, and efficient means of symptom control for many patients in the years to come.

References

1. Lip Gregory YH, Puneet K, Timothy W. Atrial fibrillation—the growing epidemic. Heart. 2007;93(5):542–3.
2. Kornej J, Borschel CP, Benjamin EJ, Schnabel RB. Epidemiology of atrial fibrillation in the 21st century: novel methods and new insights. Circ Res. 2020;127:4–20.
3. Mou L, Norby FL, Chen LY, O'Neal WT, Lewis TT, Loehr LR, Soliman EZ, Alonso A. Lifetime risk of atrial fibrillation by race and socioeconomic status: ARIC study. Circ Arrhythm Electrophysiol. 2018;11:e006350.
4. Marrouche NF, Brachmann J, Andresen D, et al. Catheter ablation for atrial fibrillation with heart failure. N Engl J Med. 2018;378:417–27.
5. Healy JS, Connolly SJ, Gold MR, et al. Subclinical atrial fibrillation and the risk of stroke. N Engl J Med. 2021;366:121–9.
6. January CT, Wann LS, et al. 2019 AHA/ACC/HRS focused update of the 2014 AHA/ACC/HRS guideline for the management of patients with atrial fibrillation: a report of the American College of Cardiology/American Heart Association Task Force on clinical practice guidelines and the Heart Rhythm Society in collaboration with the Society of Thoracic Surgeons. Circulation. 2019;140(2):e125–51.
7. Wokhlu A, et al. Long-term outcome of atrial fibrillation ablation: impact and predictors of very late recurrence. J Cardiovasc Electrophysiol. 2010;21(10):1071–8.
8. Wynn GJ, Das M, et al. Efficacy of catheter ablation for persistent atrial fibrillation: a systematic review and meta-analysis of evidence from randomized and nonrandomized controlled trials. Circ Arrhythm Electrophysiol. 2014;7(5):841–52.

9. Verma A, Jiang CY, et al. STAR AF II Investigators. Approaches to catheter ablation for persistent atrial fibrillation. N Engl J Med. 2015;372(19):1812–22.
10. Valderrábano M, Peterson LE, et al. Effect of catheter ablation with vein of Marshall ethanol infusion vs catheter ablation alone on persistent atrial fibrillation: the VENUS randomized clinical trial. JAMA. 2020;324(16):1620–8.
11. Parikh S, Jons C, Mcnitt S, et al. Predictive capability of left atrial size measured by CT, TEE and TTE for recurrence of atrial fibrillation following radiofrequency catheter ablation. PACE. 2010:1–9.
12. Kuck K-H, Brugada J, Furnkranz A, et al. Cryoballoon or radiofrequency ablation for paroxysmal atrial fibrillation. N Engl J Med. 2016;374:2235–45.
13. Andrade JG, Champagne J, Dubuc M, et al. Cryoballoon or radiofrequency ablation for atrial fibrillation assessed by continuous monitoring: a randomized clinical trial. Circulation. 2019;140(22):1779–88.
14. Bradley CJ, Haines DE. Pulsed field ablation for pulmonary vein isolation in the treatment of atrial fibrillation. J Cardiovasc Electrophysiol. 2020;31(8):2136–47.
15. Reddy VY, Dukkipati SR, Neuzil P, et al. Pulsed field ablation of paroxysmal atrial fibrillation: 1-year outcomes of IMPULSE, PEFCAT, and PEFCAT II. JACC Clin Electrophysiol. 2021;7(5):614–27.
16. Deshmukh A, Patel NJ, Pant S, et al. In-hospital complications associated with catheter ablation of atrial fibrillation in the United States between 2000 and 2010: analysis of 93 801 procedures. Circulation. 2013;128:2014–2.
17. Tripathi B, Arora S, Kumar V, et al. Temporal trends of in-hospital complications associated with catheter ablation of atrial fibrillation in the United States: an update from Nationwide Inpatient Sample database (2011–2014). J Cardiovasc Electrophysiol. 2018;29:715–24.
18. Rehman KA, Wazni OM, Barakat AF, et al. Life-threatening complications of atrial fibrillation ablation: 16-year experience in a large prospective tertiary care cohort. J Am Coll Cardiol EP. 2019;5:284–91.
19. Hall B, Jeevanantham V, Simon R, et al. Variation in left atrial transmural wall thickness at sites commonly targeted for ablation of atrial fibrillation. J Interv Card Electrophysiol. 2006;17:127–32.
20. Calkins H, Hindricks G, et al. 2017 HRS/EHRA/ECAS/APHRS/SOLAECE expert consensus statement on catheter and surgical ablation of atrial fibrillation. Heart Rhythm. 2017;14(10):e275–444.
21. Di Biase L, Burkhardt JD, et al. Periprocedural stroke and bleeding complications in patients undergoing catheter ablation of atrial fibrillation with different anticoagulation management: results from the role of coumadin in preventing thromboembolism in atrial fibrillation (AF) patients undergoing catheter ablation (COMPARE) randomized trial. Circulation. 2014;129(25):2638–44.

22. Calkins H, et al. RE-CIRCUIT study-randomized evaluation of dabigatran etexilate compared to warfarin in pulmonary vein ablation: assessment of an uninterrupted periprocedural anticoagulation strategy. Am J Cardiol. 2015;115(1):154–5.
23. Cappato R, et al. Uninterrupted rivaroxaban vs. uninterrupted vitamin K antagonists for catheter ablation in non-valvular atrial fibrillation. Eur Heart J. 2015;36(28):1805–11.
24. Kirchhof P, Haeusler KG, et al. Apixaban in patients at risk of stroke undergoing atrial fibrillation ablation. Eur Heart J. 2018;39(32):2942–55.
25. Hohnloser SH, Camm J, et al. Uninterrupted edoxaban vs. vitamin K antagonists for ablation of atrial fibrillation: the ELIMINATE-AF trial. Eur Heart J. 2019;40(36):3013–21. https://doi.org/10.1093/eurheartj/ehz190. Erratum in: Eur Heart J. 2019
26. Hussein A, Das M, Riva S, et al. Use of ablation index-guided ablation results in high rates of durable pulmonary vein isolation and freedom from arrhythmia in persistent atrial fibrillation patients. Circ Arrhythm Electrophysiol. 2018;11:e006576.
27. Das M, Loveday JJ, Wynn GJ, et al. Ablation index, a novel marker of ablation lesion quality: prediction of pulmonary vein reconnection at repeat electrophysiology study and regional differences in target values. Europace. 2017;19:775–83.
28. Das M, Duytschaever M, Gupta D, et al. Ablation index predicts sites of acute reconnection after pulmonary vein isolation: a multi-center retrospective analysis. Heart Rhythm. 2015;12:S114. Abstract
29. Ciconte G, Mugnnai G, Sieira J, et al. On the quest for the best freeze: predictors: predictors of late pulmonary vein reconnections after second-generation cryoballoon ablation. Circ Arrhythm Electrophysiol. 2015;8:1359–65.
30. Aryana A, Mugnai G, Singh SM, Pujara DK, et al. Procedural and biophysical indicators of durable pulmonary vein isolation duration cryoballoon ablation of atrial fibrillation. Heart Rhythm. 2016;13:424–32.
31. Ciconte G, Velagic V, Mugnai G, et al. Electrophysiological findings following pulmonary vein isolation using radiofrequency catheter guided by contact-force and second-generation cryoballoon: lessons from repeat procedures. Europace. 2016;18:71–7.
32. Furnkranz A, Bordignon S, Schmidt B, et al. Luminal esophageal temperature predicts esophageal lesions after second-generation cryoballoon pulmonary vein isolation. Heart Rhythm. 2013;10:789–93.
33. Metzner A, Burchard A, Wohlmuth P, et al. Increased incidence of esophageal thermal lesions using the second-generation 28-mm cryoballoon. Circ Arrhythm Electrophysiol. 2013;6:769–75.
34. Furnkranz A, Bordignon S, Bohmig M, et al. Reduced incidence of esophageal lesions by luminal esophageal temperature-guided second-generation cryoballoon ablation. Heart Rhythm. 2015;12:268–74.

35. Miyazaki S, Nakamura H, Taniguchi H, et al. Esophagus-related complications during second-generation cryoballoon ablation—insight from simultaneous esophageal temperature monitoring from 2 esophageal probes. J Cardiovasc Electrophysiol. 2016;27:1038–44.
36. Bauernfeind T, Akca F, Schwagten B, et al. The magnetic navigation system allows for safety and high efficacy for ablation of arrhythmias. Europace. 2011;13:1015–21.
37. Choi MS, Oh YS, Jang SW, et al. Comparison of magnetic navigation system and conventional method in catheter ablation of atrial fibrillation:is magnetic navigation system more effective and safer than conventional method? Korean Circ J. 2011;41:248–52.
38. Brenyo A, Rao M, Baibav B, et al. Remote magnetic navigation-guided pulmonary vein isolation: a single center experience. J Innov Card Rhythm Manag. 2013;4:1248–53.

Ventricular Tachyarrhythmias

9

Amole Ojo, Sinan Tankut, Travis Prinzi, and David T. Huang

Abstract

Ventricular tachyarrhythmias (VTAs) remain a significant contributor to the morbidity and mortality of cardiology patients population. Additionally, the incidence of VTAs are increasing in our ICD population resulting in shocks that can have a detrimental impact on quality of life. Medications alone have limited efficacy on VTAs, and can be poorly tolerated due to their side effects. The ever increasing burden and complexity of these VTAs call for novel invasive approaches for definitive treatment. Standard approaches to VT ablation such as entrainment and activation mapping remain crucial to identify the critical isthmus as a target ablation site. However, in the past decade there have been many advancements in pre-procedural imaging, mapping technologies, and approaches to substrate based ablation. Developments in techniques to epicardial ablations also allow for better procedural outcomes. Mechanical circulatory support can now be utilized among tenuous patients and allows for safer and more precise ablations. There are also

A. Ojo (✉) · S. Tankut · T. Prinzi · D. T. Huang
University of Rochester Medical Center, Rochester, NY, USA
e-mail: Amole_Ojo@urmc.Rochester.edu

non-invasive treatments for refractory VTAs not responsive to medical therapy or amenable to catheter ablation. In this chapter, we review the different mechanisms of VTAs, medical treatments, advancements in mapping technologies and approaches to catheter ablation, and discuss non-invasive treatments for VTAs.

Keywords

Ventricular tachyarrhthmia · Ventricular tachycardia · Ventricular fibrillation · Electroanatomic mapping · Activation mapping · Entrainment mapping · Catheter ablation · Epicardial access · Substrate modification · Cardiac radioablation

Introduction

Ventricular tachyarrhythmias can present with a wide variety of symptoms, including sudden cardiac death. There are several causes of sustained arrhythmias that originate from the ventricles and can have varying prognosis and therapy needs to be tailored accordingly. Understanding critical aspects of ventricular arrhythmias such as initiating mechanisms, proper risk stratification and response to medical and ablation therapies is critical in the proper treatment of the patients with these conditions.

How Do Arrhythmias Start?

Electrical impulse normally travels through the heart chambers in a very organized and uniform manner. However, disturbances in how electrical signals are initiated or how they propagate through the cardiac chamber can lead to the onset of arrhythmias. In general, there are three mechanisms of how arrhythmias start. A common arrhythmia mechanism is impulse reentry. Tissues may intrinsically exhibit multiple pathways (as in dual atrioventricular nodal physiology, see "Chap. 3, SVT") or develop multiple pathways in the healing process (as in scars post myocardial infarction) through which the electrical signal may travel. If these paths are associated with different conduction velocities and correspondingly different refractory periods, the electrical signals can circle around in an "endless loop" through these circuit paths. Conditions suitable for reentry require the slower conducting pathway to have a shorter refractory period and the faster conducting pathway to have a longer refractory period. Most ventricular tachycardias (VT), though certainly not all, related to post myocardial infarction substrate or cardiomyopathy are due to impulse reentry. Monomorphic VT is often due to stable and fixed circuits of reentry whereas polymorphic VT can be due to unstable and meandering or even multiple circuits of reentry. Another mechanism for arrhythmia onset is due to triggered activity. Increased intracellular calcium concentration due to heightened adrenergic stimulation (such as exercise), initiates a cascade of reaction through activation of stimulatory G proteins resulting in enhanced calcium entry through the cellular calcium channels and calcium induced calcium release in the sarcoplasmic reticulum. This increase in the intracellular calcium then may activate the sodium calcium exchanger leading to abnormal sodium entry into the cell which may trigger depolarization of the heart cell resulting in premature beats or even tachycardia [1]. Forms of normal heart idiopathic ventricular tachycardia associated with exercise, such as one originating right ventricular outflow tract, are often resulting from triggered activity. A third mechanism for arrhythmogenesis is enhanced automaticity, where cardiac muscle tissue develops spontaneous electrical activity through abnormal depolarization during phase 4 of the action potential. These arrhythmias are usually referred as "automatic" tachycardia. Some examples of these include variants of tachycardia related to diseased tissue where the baseline membrane potential may be unstable. Typically, sources of tachycardia that are focal are due to either triggered activity or enhanced automaticity.

The management of ventricular arrhythmias is thus complex and quite variable, with this variance discussed in the following segments. Our initial focus will be scar mediated VT (VT with an abnormal left ventricular ejection fraction [LVEF]) followed by idiopathic PVC's and less frequent forms of idiopathic ventricular tachycardia (VT with a normal LVEF).

Electrocardiographic Evaluation of Ventricular Arrhythmias

The first and most important diagnostic tool remains the 12 lead electrocardiogram during a wide QRS complex tachycardia. Often the type of cardiomyopathy, location of scarring, and VT exit can be estimated from the appearance of the tachycardia. Multiple algorithms have been developed and studied for the electrocardiographic diagnosis of VT including the Brugada criteria [2] and various individual lead (Lead II, AVR) [3, 4] analysis techniques all with good specificity and sensitivity for the identification of VT in distinction from supraventricular tachyarrhythmias (SVT) with aberrancy. All these algorithms take advantage of the initial forces of activation to distinguish VT from SVT. Tachycardia of ventricular origin depolarized the myocardial muscles by cell-to-cell contact and thus will have slower forces of activation represented by delayed or fragmented portions early in the QRS signals. On the other hand, during SVT, even with aberrancy, the heart muscles are activated via engaging the specialized conduction tissues and are generally associated with a more smooth and rapid initial QRS signals. Of note, all of these algorithms are qualified and should be used with caution in patients with manifest preexcitation (i.e., Wolff-Parkinson-White syndrome) or on antiarrhythmic medical therapy. Updated morphology criteria developed in recent years have more elegant and simplified algorithm to decipher whether a wide complex tachycardia may be VT or SVT with aberrancy. Inspecting the morphology of the initial QRS signals in lead aVR can be used to suggest ventricular origin of a wide complex tachycardia. As illustrated in Fig. 9.1, QRS with slow or notched initial forces as well as those with unusual axis all suggest a diagnosis of VT rather than SVT. Similarly, if the duration of the QRS signal from the beginning of the onset to the peak of the R wave in lead II measures to be greater or equal

9 Ventricular Tachyarrhythmias

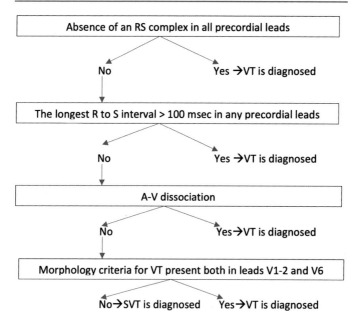

Fig. 9.1 Algorithm to determine VT vs. SVT with aberrancy as described by Brugada et al. [2]

to 50 msec, then VT can be diagnosed with better than 95% confidence (Figs. 9.1, 9.2 and 9.3).

Once diagnosis is made that the arrhythmia is VT, the next step is to determine the activation vector of the ventricle. As a simplistic starting point, the bundle branch block appearance of the QRS complex indicates the culprit chamber where the VT is originating from. A left bundle branch block appearance indicates an RV or septal LV VT while a right bundle branch appearance indicates an LV VT origin. Taking this approach a step further, using the right sided leads (V1, AVR), inferior leads (II/III/AVF), lateral leads (1/AVL) and apical leads (V5/V6) one can identify where the VT is coming from (negative QS vector) and going towards (positive RS vector). Generally, biphasic QRS vectors mean that the origin is somewhere in the middle of that individual vector, i.e. a biphasic QRS vector in 1 and V1 likely indicate that the origin/exit site of

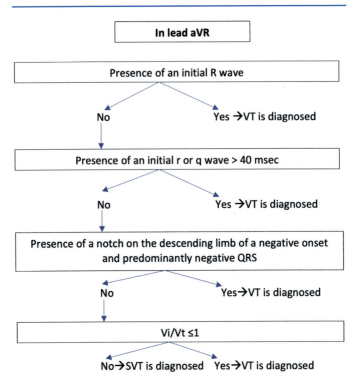

Fig. 9.2 Algorithm to determine VT vs. SVT with aberrancy by criteria developed in lead aVR [3]

the VT is in the septum and not on the right (RV, Q wave in V1) or left (posterior LV, Q wave in 1). This approach is primarily useful in reentrant VT's and idiopathic PVC's.

A close examination of the resting 12 lead ECG can also provide significant clues as to the underlying process and likely culprit areas of myocardial scarring. The presence of Q waves in the distribution of a coronary artery should indicate the presence of scarring that will often play a critical role in sustaining VT. Fragmentation (extra notching) of the surface QRS complex in a similar distribution to a major coronary vessel and Q waves

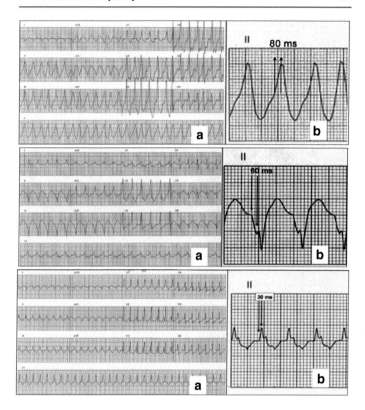

Fig. 9.3 Algorithm to determine VT vs. SVT by measuring the duration of onset of QRS to the peak of R wave lead II (**a** - 12 lead ECG; **b** - lead II). Signals measuring >50 msec (top two panels) suggest VT whereas <50 ms suggest SVT with aberrancy [4]

often can provide a more sensitive indicator of myocardial scarring and may indicate the presence of epicardial scarring in that region. There are also ECG criterias to help differentiate endocardial versus epicardial VT. The maximum deflection index is a ratio from the beginning of the QRS to the maximum deflection point to the total width of the QRS. If the ratio is ≥0.55, idiopathic left ventricular VT was likely to be epicardial in origin [5]. Other published morphology criteria include q wave in lead I (QWLI) and no q waves in inferior leads and interval criteria: pseudo-delta wave ≥34 ms, intrinsicoid deflection time ≥ 85 ms, and shortest RS complex ≥121 ms.

For idiopathic VT's such as RVOT and LVOT VT, the appearance should be consistent with an outflow origin (inferior axis, i.e., positive in the inferior leads II/III/AVF) with an earlier precordial transition (V3 or less) indicating an LV origin and a later transition (V3 or later) indicating an RV origin. Transition at V3 could represent either LV or RV origin. V2 transition ratio can help to distinguish LVOT origin from RVOT origin in patients with lead V3 precordial transition. V2 transition ratio is calculated by computing the percentage R-wave during VT (R/R + S)(VT) divided by the percentage R-wave in sinus rhythm (R/R + S)(SR). In a study by Betensky et al., a V(2) transition ratio ≥ 0.60 predicted an LVOT origin with 91% accuracy while a PVC precordial transition occurring later than the sinus rhythm transition excluded an LVOT origin with 100% accuracy [6]. RV1-V3 transition ratio is another criterion that can be used to distinguish LVOT from RVOT origin in patients with lead V3 precordial transition. RV1-V3 is defined as (RV1 + RV2 + RV3) PVC / (RV1 + RV2 + RV3) SR (sinus rhythm). In the study by Efremidis et al., a cut-off value of ≥0.9 predicting LVOT origin with 94% sensitivity and 73% specificity [7]. Idiopathic VT utilizing the conduction system (bundle branch and fasicular reentry VT's) are quite uncommon but do have characteristic features that should set them aside from VT associated with structural heart disease. The VT is generally slower with a typical bundle branch or fasicular block appearance during tachycardia that is usually very similar to the appearance of the baseline QRS complex at rest. Bundle branch and fasicular reentry are usually associated with baseline conduction disease, including bundle branch block of either right or left and prolonged AV or PR interval, with the absence of such on a resting 12 lead ECG making them very unlikely to be the mechanism for the VT.

Scar Mediated Ventricular Tachycardia

Within westernized cultures the most common underlying cause of recurrent VT is remote coronary disease. Secondary to a focus on shorter door to balloon times for the acute myocardial infarction patients, more patients are surviving their myocardial infarctions only to eventually experience downstream congestive heart failure and ventricular tachycardia. The ischemic insult of a myocardial infarction results in the formation of myocardial scarring with variable transmural extent and resulting in altered electrical conduction within the infracted myocardial region. Electrical conduction through scar is delayed and the resultant zone of slow conduction represents one of the critical elements of the reentrant circuit. This along with differential refractory periods in the surrounding tissue comprise the necessary substrate to sustain VT [8]. Ventricular ectopy often is the inciting event that initiates the ventricular tachyarrhythmia, either VT or VF. Premature ventricular contractions are sent through the slow conduction zone present within the ventricular scar with sufficient delay to result in their exit on the opposite side of the scarred region finding the myocardium ready for depolarization. The electrical wave propagates around the more dense areas of scarring or anatomical barrier such as heart valve annulus and back into the entrance of the zone of slow conduction through the scar creating a figure of eight pattern with the critical isthmus representing the central portion of the figure of eight (Fig. 9.4).

The typical ischemic ventricular tachycardia patient will present to medical care with either recurrent defibrillator therapies (shocks) or recurrent presyncope. Presyncope VT patients, with transvenous implantable cardioverter-defibrillator (ICD), are often being treated with antitachycardia pacing (ATP) and thus being prevented from progressing to either shocks or actual syncope. ATP works by delivering appropriately timed sequential ventricular pacing into an excitable gap during a reentrant circuit, such as ventricular tachycardia [9]. Studies have demonstrated ATP to be safe, painless, and effective at treating ventricular arrhythmias, including fast VT [10]. Burst pacing allows a fixed

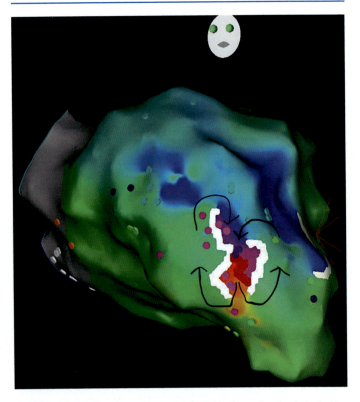

Fig. 9.4 Figure of eight reentrant ventricular tachycardia circuit encircling around a dense anteroseptal left ventricular scar. The central portion of the figure of eight comprises the critical isthmus with a zone of slow conduction and the area where diastolic potentials may be recorded. This site, following confirmation with pacing maneuvers, often is the target of successful ablation

RR interval to be delivered (usually with a coupling interval of 84–88% of the tachycardia cycle length) with a set amount of stimulus delivered, varying from 8–12 beats. Ramp pacing is an ATP mode that delivers ventricular stimulus in a sequential, decremental fashion starting at selected RR interval (8–12 beats). Scan is an ATP mode when the pacing cycle length is shortened between each pacing train. All ATP modes have demonstrated to be effective in terminating VT and are a programmable option for all major device companies. iATP is a feature which gives customized ATP in real time in some device companies. An iATP algorithm delivers the equivalent of a train of Burst pulses (S1) followed by 1 (S2) or 2 (S2-S3) extra- stimuli Ramp+ pulses. The protocol for the first iATP sequence is S1-S2. If the first sequence does not terminate the tachyarrhythmia, the protocol for the subsequent sequences is S1-S2 or S1-S2-S3. If patients are hemodynamically stable and manual ATP to be performed, it is recommended that patients receive sedation as delivery of ATP can result in the degeneration of ventricular tachycardia to ventricular fibrillation requiring emergent ICD or external electrical shock. Of concern is the patient that presents with incessant VT or frequent, defined as >3 episodes of VT within 24 hours, termed VT storm often requiring multiple shocks and acute inpatient admission for management accompanied by a significant rise in both inpatient and short term mortality [11]. The management of all of these patients is similar with a few exceptions made for the VT storm patient. In general, recurrent antitachycardia pacing or lone outpatient ICD shocks should result in the initiation or acceleration of antiarrhythmic drug therapy starting with sotalol or amiodarone followed by the addition of mexiletine if necessary. It is also important to make sure that these patients are adequately beta blocked since the majority of ischemic VT's are going to possess an adrenergic component and be beneficially treated with beta blockade. Catheter ablation for ventricular tachycardia has traditionally been viewed as a last resort or palliative treatment for ventricular arrhythmias. However, with significant developments in mapping systems, improvement in diagnostic and therapeutic ablation catheters, along with the ability to hemodynamically support patients with mechanical circulatory support, catheter ablation for VT are being utilized earlier in the treatment course of patients. Hence, it is reasonable to consider VT ablation instead of initiation of antiarrhythmic medication in the management of these patients even following first VT event. Once patients experience recurrent ICD therapies for VT while on an appropriate antiarrhythmic drug regimen, ventricular tachycardia ablation should absolutely be considered.

The management of VT storm patients is more difficult and varied than the ambulatory cardiomyopathy patients with recurrent ATP or lone ICD shocks for ventricular tachycardia. VT storm patients present with recurrent ICD shocks often are accompanied by hemodynamic instability. The first step in their management is to establish control of their ventricular rhythm. Intravenous antiarrhythmic agents are utilized acutely to achieve this with both amiodarone and lidocaine used commonly. Although limited by toxicity, lidocaine can be a useful agent especially if there are concerns for ongoing ischemia. However, a combination of amiodarone (or sotalol) and lidocaine is often required to achieve control of the malignant ventricular arrhythmias in this situation. In addition to antiarrhythmic drug therapy and aggressive beta blockade, sedation and sometimes intubation are utilized to minimize adrenergic contribution to the VT. As an illustrative point to the contribution of sympathetic tone to the generation of recurrent VT in patients with an abnormal LVEF, bilateral sympathectomy has been shown to be effective for the suppression of acute ICD therapies for VT storm patients and has displayed durability over medium term follow up [12]. During VT storm, Stellate ganglion nerve blocks in conjunction with intravenous antiarrhythmic use can help stabilize ventricular arrhythmias.

Following the initiation of intravenous antiarrhythmic drug therapy, ongoing myocardial ischemia should be considered and evaluated, likely with coronary angiography. If myocardial ischemia is present and is the main substrate of the VT, successful treatment with revascularization often subsides the VT. However, it is usually required to accelerate the patient's oral antiarrhythmic drug therapy prior to discharge and to establish short term follow up to make sure that the treated lesion was indeed the ischemic driver of the VT.

For VT storm patients or ambulatory patients with recurrent VT despite antiarrhythmic drug therapy, electrophysiologic testing and ablation of their VT should be considered. VT ablation has evolved since its inception to a well defined repeatable process designed to identify electrical scar, the culprit ventricular tachycardia and its dependent isthmus.

Electrophysiologic Evaluation of VT with Structural Heart Disease

Twelve lead ECGs can provide a general idea of the origin of the VT. However, lead displacement and other pitfalls from localizing arrhythmias from a 12 lead ECG cannot be solely used for pre-procedural planning. Various imaging modalities can be used to help further identify scar, inflammation, or areas of infiltrative disease that can support the localization of VT in preparation for VT ablation. The use of cardiac CT, MRI, and nuclear imaging can help identify the location of the arrhythmic substrate to assist in intraprocedural mapping. Furthermore, information from pre-procedural imaging can also help assist if epicardial access will be needed during the procedure. Current guidelines give a class I recommendation to obtain pre procedural imaging to rule out a cardiac thrombi to reduce the risk of catheter induced thromboembolic events [13]. The most cost effective and practical option is obtaining a transthoracic echocardiogram with visualization of cardiac chambers with echo contrast.

Yamashita et al. studied the effectiveness of image integration with procedural mapping for scar related ventricular tachycardia. Imaging with either multi-detector computed tomography (MDCT) and late gadolinium-enhancement cardiac magnetic resonance (LGE-CMR) were obtained 1–3 days prior to planned catheter ablation. The images were processed using the MUSIC software and the results from the study showed that the arrhythmic substrate obtained from imaging correlated with local abnormal ventricular activity and the critical isthmus [14]. The ability to localize the VT substrate and potential ablation sites on imaging can decrease duration of the procedure and improve outcomes.

For patients being evaluated for EP testing and ablation of a ventricular arrhythmia it is important to provide the appropriate setting. The use of general anesthesia for these procedures has become standard secondary to the length of the procedure and the risk for multiple defibrillations. However, there is still role for monitored anesthesia care when there is concern that patient's VT may become hemodynamically unstable following administration of general anesthesia. Three dimensional mapping systems have also become standard and represent one of the most powerful tools to allow an in depth study of the ventricular chamber in question and increase the efficacy of VT ablation.

Prior to the procedure, the patient should be thoroughly assessed regarding the appropriate approach to the chamber in question. Generally the right ventricle does not pose much of a challenge outside of patients with complex congenital heart disease or tricuspid valve surgery. However the left ventricle may prove inaccessible from a retroaortic or transseptal approach due to the presence of mechanical aortic or mitral valves. The location of culprit scar is also an important consideration as anterior and basal septal walls are more easily accessible from a transseptal approach while LVOT, apex, inferior, and lateral walls are via a retroaortic approach. Peripheral arterial disease can make a retroaortic approach difficult if not impossible which should prompt the performance of a peripheral arterial exam (bruits and pulses) prior to procedure onset. In addition, the ability to access the epicardial space (the absence of a prior sternotomy) should also be considered at procedure onset to determine if it is an option if required.

During procedure onset and throughout the duration, control of the patient's bradyarrhythmia should be available through the implanted device (in the likely event that it is present). It is best to leave patients that are not ventricular pacing dependent paced in the atrium only to allow intrinsic conduction for more accurate endocardial scar mapping. For ventricular pacing dependent patients it is often necessary to leave biventricular pacing in place to maintain appropriate hemodynamic status for the purpose of anesthesia. It may also be necessary to review the induced ventricular tachycardia on the far field electrogram through the device, which is only possible if the programmer is on and communicating with the device. The implanted device can also provide a means of intracardiac defibrillation if such a rescue is needed.

Once access to the LV endocardium or epicardium has been obtained, electrophysiolic study and ablation of ventricular tachycardia proceeds in four steps: (1) anatomic definition; (2) endocardial scar mapping; (3) induction and study of ventricular tachycardia, including entrainment mapping; (4) ablation of ventricular tachycardia, late potentials within scar; (5) attempt reinduction of ventricular tachycardia. With abolition of the clinical ventricular tachycardia and inability to induce anything other than ventricular fibrillation or polymorphic VT, the study is complete.

To define the left ventricular anatomy a three dimensional map is generated with the aid of either fluoroscopy or ultrasound and often both. Other than the geometry of the left ventricule itself, this often includes structures such as the mitral annulus, left ventricular outflow tract, left sided His bundle, Purkinje potentials and papillary muscles. It is important to make sure that the anatomy collected is complete. Correspondingly, the right ventricular structures including the AV node and the His conduction system, tricuspid valve, pulmonic valve, right ventricular outflow tract should be noted. Generally the risk of right ventricular perforation is higher and thus more care during mapping is needed. As the definition of endocardial scarring is dependent upon catheter contact with the wall, it is essential to know if contact is indeed present, otherwise areas will be labeled as scar inappropriately. This has been aided with real time two dimensional intracardiac echocardiography along with the evolution of contact force catheters which both can be used to provide definitive evidence of endocardial contact. Multi-electrode mapping catheters are commonly utilized to collect a significantly larger amount of data in a shorter period of time both regarding anatomy and endocardial voltage.

Generally at the same time that anatomic information is collected, voltage is collected to provide visual information of the distribution of endocardial scarring relative to the anatomy collected. The definition of endocardial scar varies somewhat but is generally accepted to be any myocardial tissue with less than 0.5 mv. In similar fashion to the necessity of complete anatomic collection, it is just as important to generate a complete detailed voltage map. With identification of the scar, additional focus should be placed upon the scar itself for either fragmented potentials or late potentials coined to be local abnormal ventricular activities or LAVA. LAVA are characterized by high frequency or fragmented signals that can be either late relative to the QRS com-

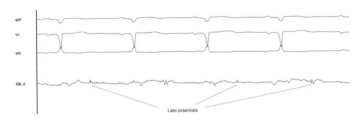

Fig. 9.5 Late systolic potentials noted during substrate ventricular mapping recorded in sinus rhythm

plex and local signal or buried completely within the local signal (Fig. 9.5).

In addition, areas that LV capture may be generated from within the endocardial scar are suspicious for possible VT isthmus and should be tagged for eventual ablation.

With a complete endocardial scar map, the next step within our lab is to induce ventricular tachycardia via programmed stimulation via a quadripolar pacing catheter in the RV. A predominantly substrate based approach does not involve induction of VT and ablation is carried out with the intention to abolish all LAVA within and around the endocardial scar. At this point it is crucial to reference the tachycardia 12-lead ECG for the rate and appearance of the VT, if available. Within the defibrillator population one may not ever have a surface electrocardiogram as the majority of their events are treated prior to presentation to medical care via their device. As a result only the cycle length and far field electrogram through the device are available to correlate the VT induced during the procedure with the clinical VT.

Once VT is induced matching the clinical VT the approach to study of the VT can vary from patient to patient. If the VT is hemodynamically tolerable (most often seen with slower VT's [<150 bpm] in patients with only moderate LV dysfunction) then activation and entrainment mapping may be pursued. If not hemodynamically tolerable, then the VT is pace terminated or terminated via defibrillation and pace mapping to define the VT isthmus based upon the VT morphology followed by a LAVA ablation strategy is appropriate. Both situations will be discussed in the following sections.

The Study of Hemodynamically Tolerable VT

Hemodynamically tolerable VT has become increasingly uncommon within the electrophysiology lab. Most of the VT's that are being mapped currently are fast VT's in patients with more advanced LV dysfunction. It may often be necessary to utilize vasopressors or in some cases device based hemodynamic support (Intra-aortic balloon pump, percutaneous left ventricular assist device such as Impella or ECMO) to provide adequate perfusion pressure in an effort to allow mapping. Goal blood pressures should be a mean arterial pressure above 60 mmHg.

When VT is tolerable it is beneficial to perform activation and entrainment mapping to confidently abolish the clinical VT. Points are taken and recorded via the mapping system to identify early and late EGM's with the area in the scar connecting early to late representing the slow component of the VT circuit and the critical isthmus. Within the early meets late area entrainment via the mapping catheter is performed by pacing 10–20 ms faster than the VT. Capture is maintained for sufficient time to overtake the VT circuit (5–10 beats) followed by cessation. If the morphology of the tachycardia changes during pacing, termed "manifest entrainment", and is associated with a post pacing interval (PPI) longer than the tachycardia cycle length then the pacing site is from an area outside of the tachycardia circuit (remote bystander). Ablation at these sites will not result in termination of VT. Suitable targets for successful ablation should result in "concealed entrainment". Pacing from these sites result in acceleration and exact morphology match as the tachycardia. Sites associated with the highest short and long term success in eliminating the VT circuit with ablation are in the critical isthmus. In addition to concealed entrainment, pacing from within the critical isthmus, the difference between the PPI and the tachycardia cycle length (TCL) will be small (less than 30 msec) plus recording of presystolic potentials with an activation time to surface QRS similar to stimulus to surface QRS (less than 20 msec) indicate that the mapping catheter is located within the VT critical isthmus (Fig. 9.6). Ablation at this site typically at 30-45 watts with an irrigated ablation catheter should result in the termination of VT promptly (Figs. 9.7, 9.8 and 9.9).

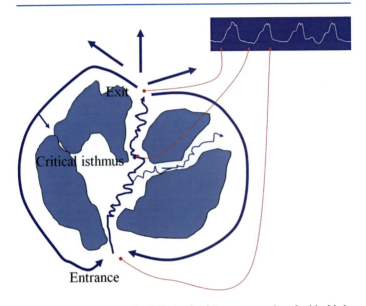

Fig. 9.6 Diagram illustrating VT circuit with entrance, exit and critical isthmus sites denoted

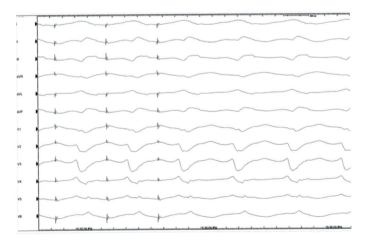

Fig. 9.7 Pacing from the critical isthmus of the VT circuit resulting in "concealed entrainment" with 12 out of 12 lead surface ECG match in pacing morphology as compared with VT morphology

9 Ventricular Tachyarrhythmias 197

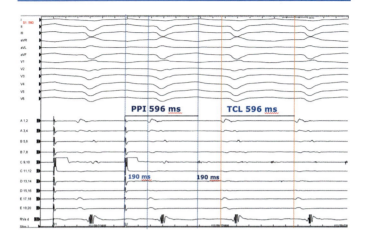

Fig. 9.8 Other criteria for pacing within the critical isthmus of the VT circuit with pacing stimulus to QRS = EGM to QRS and post pacing interval (PPI) equal to VT cycle length

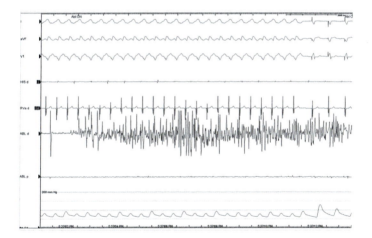

Fig. 9.9 Ablation at the critical isthmus site results in termination of VT

In some cases the isthmus is wide and some catheter manipulation is required to completely transect the isthmus. Following thorough ablation of the isthmus (noncapture of the targeted region with high output pacing via the mapping catheter), the culprit VT should be rendered non-inducible. Once found to be non-inducible, scar modification via targeting of LAVA is usually undertaken to improve the long term success of the VT ablation and hopefully prevent subsequent VT's. This approach will be discussed in the third and final study/ablation approach.

The Study of Hemodynamically Unstable VT

In recent years, peri-procedural mechanical circulatory support has been utilized in patients with known hemodynamically unstable VTs in order to perform both activation and entrainment mapping [15]. Ablation of hemodynamically unstable VT can still be performed even without mechanical circulatory support. In such cases, induction of hemodynamically unstable VT should be followed by termination of the VT either via pacing or defibrillation. The VT is then reviewed with the vector of the VT QRS utilized to identify the exit site from the identified endocardial scar. At this stage pace mapping with a software based match typically provided via the 3D mapping system to the induced VT is used to identify the exit (best match, generally >90% in 12 leads, ideally >95% match) and entrance (worst match) with the isthmus connecting the two. Entrance and exit are usually spatially related as the length of the typical VT isthmus is usually 20–30 mm and with detailed pace mapping can be readily identified. This isthmus is transsected with thorough ablation rendering the targeted area not able to be captured with pacing and the VT should be rendered non-inducible. Following abolition of the clinical VT additional scar modification is generally performed similar to that following successful entrainment and activation guided VT ablation.

Substrate Modification for VT

Scar modification or homogenization has been utilized as a primary approach for patients with unstable VT's or multiple VT's and is often performed after successful abolition of the culprit clinical VT. With detailed scar mapping, LAVA are targeted with the goal of elimination of the late potential. A more diffuse approach can also be taken where the entire scar is ablated or linear transsecting lesions are placed through the scar or the scar is circumscribed with contiguous ablation. Areas with the ability to capture the LV within the scar are also common targets for scar modification. The major downside of this as a primary approach is the uncertainty regarding successful treatment of the culprit clinical VT. Of the strategies available: LAVA, linear lesions, abolition of pacing capture or scar isolation, the selected strategy is often dependent upon the location and size of the scar accompanied by the comfort level of the performing physician. Recent data supports favorable results following LAVA guided scar homogenization however it is not always possible to completely eliminate every LAVA within the scar which may make the use of a more diffuse strategy an appropriate backup measure. High density mapping can also help to identify deceleration zones. Isochronal late activation mapping (ILAM) is performed during sinus rhythm or ventricular paced rhythm to identify the deceleration zones. The latest local electrocardiograms are utilized. Area of deceleration zones are defined as >3 isochrones within 1 cm radius. Tung et al. performed VT ablations on 120 patients using deceleration zones as the target ablation site. After a mean 12 month follow up period, 70% of patients did not have recurrence of VT [16].

Epicardial Mapping

Often when one is unable to successfully eradicate the culprit VT via endocardial mapping and ablation, the consideration of epicardial mapping follows. Also, epicardial mapping should be considered especially in patients with non-ischemic cardiomyopathy and also when 12 lead ECG of the VT is suggestive of epicardial origin. It is important to consider this option when discussing the procedure with the patient to make sure that the risks of this approach are understood. Prior cardiac surgery makes this significantly more difficult and should serve as a relative contraindication to this approach.

Our approach is to obtain epicardial access via a dry pericardial tap; a subxyphoid approach is generally utilized with the area prepped and draped as per routine to start. A Tuohy needle is utilized and advanced under the skin and the rib cage toward the left shoulder, oriented according to the targeted ventricular surface (i.e., anterior, shallow <45° vs. inferior, steep >45°) under fluoroscopy. The glide wire present within the needle can be advanced intermittently to see if the needle has found the pericardial space. Once the wire enters the pericardial space it should be advanced aggressively to wrap the entire outline of the pericardium in multiple loops. A subxiphoid puncture should ideally be performed before administration of systemic anticoagulation. Epicardial access can still be safely obtained in patients on heparin However, reversal with protamine to aim for an activated clotting time of <200 sec is recommended, whenever possible. Our epicardial access approach has changed to needle-in-needle technique. A smaller 21-gauge, 15- and/or 20-cm long micropuncture needle is used to assess the pericardium. To provide stability, the micropuncture needle is inserted through a standard 7-cm, 18-gauge access needle or a Tuohy needle. Once the needle reaches the pericardium, cardiac pulsations can be felt. A small amount of contrast can be given at this point and this will indicate the location of the needle tip. If contrast injection results in staining of the pericardial fat or the pericardium, the needle may be slowly advanced another 1 to 2 mm and contrast injection repeated until the pericardium is accessed. The puncture of the fibrous pericardium may be accompanied by a noticeable "pop" and appreciated with the release of resistance on the needle. A small injection of contrast should result in diffuse dispersion of contrast throughout the pericardium and along the cardiac silhouette. If the RV has been penetrated, there will be rapid washout of the contrast. In this case, the needle should be withdrawn slightly while reinject-

9 Ventricular Tachyarrhythmias

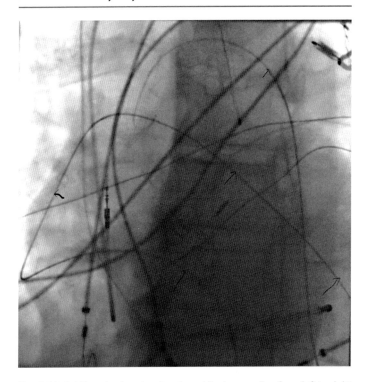

Fig. 9.10 LAO projection showing the guidewire crossing from left to right across multiple cardiac chambers. Arrows point to the course of the guidewire

ing a small amount of contrast until the pericardium is entered. Once pericardial access is obtained using the micropuncture needle, a 0.018- inch long guidewire is advanced into the pericardium, which is subsequently exchanged for a standard 0.032-inch long guidewire to allow insertion of larger bore epicardial introducers. The position of the guidewire must be validated in the LAO projection. The wire must always be visualized following the left heart border and crossing unrestrictedly from the left to the right, anterior to the great vessels (Fig. 9.10).

Once the wire is in place, a short steerable epicardial sheath is advanced over the wire into the pericardial space. Following this, anatomic and voltage/scar mapping using a multi electrode or ablation catheter can proceed in the same fashion as endocardial mapping. Entrainment and pace mapping can be performed similar to the endocardium as well with the major limiting factor being the ability to capture the LV due to the presence of epicardial fat in areas. It is always important to define coronary anatomy via coronary angiography with the ablation catheter in the area of desired ablation prior to ablation in an effort to not directly ablate a major epicardial vessel. Another consideration before delivering epicardial ablation lesions is the course of the left phrenic nerve. The left phrenic nerve descends over the fibrous pericardium along either: (1) the lateral margin of the LV (59%) or a posterior-inferior direction (23%); or (2) the anterior surface of the LV (18%) [17]. Injury can be avoided with precautionary measures such as high-output pacing (ϵ10 mA) when ablating within the territory of the left phrenic nerve. Alternatively, the phrenic nerve may be protected from the path of radiofrequency energy by injecting air and/or saline into the pericardial space or simply by positioning a balloon catheter between the ablation site and the phrenic nerve. Once the scar has been mapped and the isthmus defined to be within a safe region ablation is generally performed at 25–35 watts via an irrigated ablation catheter.

With a complete ablation within the pericardium a pigtail drain is exchanged for the steerable sheath over wire with the drain left in place overnight if the aspirated fluid is bloody. If the aspirated fluid is clear, there is no need to leave a drain overnight. Prior to removal of the sheath or drain, our practice is to infuse corticosteroids (Solumedrol, triamcinolone or hydrocortisone) within the pericardial space to minimize the risk of subsequent pericarditis.

Electrophysiologic Evaluation of Idiopathic VT

There is a well-defined category of VT seen in patients who are typically younger without structural or ischemic cardiovascular disease. Outflow tract VT's and high burden PVC's are the predominant arrhythmias encountered within this category. These normal heart VT's may originate from the outflow tract and some originate from the inferoposterior septal LV, termed as fascicular

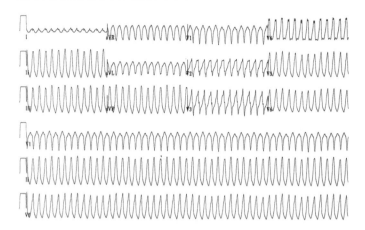

Fig. 9.11 Twelve lead ECG of a patient with ventricular tachycardia originating from the right ventricular outflow tract. Note the typical left bundle branch block morphology with inferior QRS axis as well as the large R wave amplitudes in the inferior leads

or "Belhassen" variant VT. It is important to have a clinical suspicion for these less common VT's as the procedural approach to their electrophysiologic study and treatment is quite different from VT with structural cardiovascular disease. VT's originating from the outflow tracts typically have an inferior axis with large R wave amplitudes in the inferior leads (Fig. 9.11).

The morphology of the idiopathic inferoposterior septal LV VT is consistent with typical right bundle branch block pattern with an LAFB axis (Fig. 9.12).

Outflow tract VT's, especially those originating from the right ventricular regions are well understood to be due to triggered activity and are generally responsive to beta blockade and calcium channel blockade medical therapy. On the other hand, fascicular or "Belhassen VT" has also been coined "Verapamil Sensitive VT" because its mechanism is thought be due to a small circuit reentry in the inferoposterior septum that is calcium dependent. Often invasive electrophysiologic study and ablation are reserved for medical treatment failures with these agents.

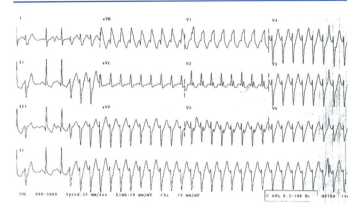

Fig. 9.12 Twelve lead ECG of a patient with an idiopathic normal heart ventricular tachycardia originating from the left ventricular inferoposterior septum. Note the right bundle branch block morphology with superior QRS axis

For patients with symptomatic idiopathic PVC's, the majority of the clinical decision making centers around the burden of PVC's and their location. A PVC burden of at least 10% or greater on ambulatory monitoring is considered high volume and at risk for developing subsequent PVC induced LV dysfunction. PVC origins within the RVOT are lowest risk for PVC cardiomyopathy with any LV location being higher risk for downstream LV functional decline. In addition, PVC's with a QRS duration of greater than 150 ms are also high risk for LV dyssynchrony and if frequent enough volume can cause LV dysfunction.

Medical therapy via beta blockade alone often may result in some reduction in the PVC burden but some patients may still be left with high burden PVC's and at risk for cardiomyopathy even on medical therapy. Antiarrhythmic drug therapy via Class 1 (flecainide, propafenone, mexiletine) or Class III (sotalol, amiodarone) may result in a further reduction in PVC burden which may be utilized as adjunctive therapy for patients with high volume PVC's. Once on medical therapy, PVC burden should be reassessed with repeat ambulatory monitoring to make sure that the PVC burden on therapy is low enough to preclude the development of PVC induced cardiomyopathy. Persistence of high burden PVC's or symptoms despite antiarrhythmic drug therapy should prompt consideration for electrophysiologic study and ablation of the PVC focus. The presence of multiform PVC's or non-outflow tract locations are risk factors for requiring multiple procedures to effectively reduce the PVC burden which should be discussed with the patient prior to proceeding.

Electrophysiologic Testing and Ablation of Idiopathic PVC's and Outflow Tract VT's

After medical treatment failure or in patients unwilling to attempt medical therapy, electrophysiologic testing with an eye to ablation therapy for those with documented outflow tract VT or high burden idiopathic PVC's is appropriate. Of note, these procedures generally do not require general anesthesia and are best approached with as little sedation as possible secondary to a reduction in PVC burden associated with aggressive sedation. Without spontaneous PVC's it is difficult to confidently map and eliminate the PVC. Isuprel, atropine, aminophylline and programmed stimulation from either the RV apex or outflow tract are often utilized. Generally outflow tract patients have single outflow tract PVC's that represent the source of their more sustained episodes of VT. Mapping and ablation of these PVC's usually treat their sustained VT. For PVC patients it is important to determine their triggers. If their PVC's come out when they are resting, sedation may be appropriate; in contrast if they are associated with caffeine, isoproterenol may be appropriate, etc.

The PVC morphology is captured once the patient is on the table and logged within the 3D mapping system for comparison should pace mapping be utilized. Usually QRS morphology can be used to identify location of the PVC (LVOT or RVOT) with the precordial transition being the most usefull but imperfect tool. R/S transition prior to V3 can confidently be labeled as LVOT with a transition after V3 labeled as RVOT. The use of multielectrode mapping catheters for both anatomic, pacing and activation mapping can make identification of the PVC focus easier. Once in

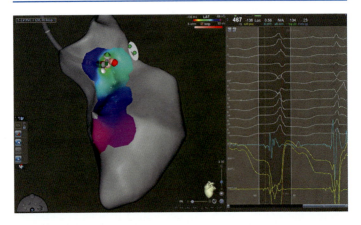

Fig. 9.13 A small prepotential is seen on the ablation catheter in the LVOT preceeding the onset of the QRS

the appropriate location anatomy is collected first with particular attention to details such as the His bundle on the RV side and the aortic cusp/coronary anatomy on the LV side. Ultrasound can be of great use for aortic and LVOT PVC's/VT to minimize the risk of damage to sensitive structures such as the ostium of the left or right coronary arteries.

With anatomy collected, the preferential modality is activation mapping of spontaneous PVC's focusing on only including PVC's that are completely consistent with the clinical PVC and not catheter induced. Once the area of activation is narrowed down sufficiently the exact area should be able to be identified usually with a small pre potential prior to the larger local EGM on the mapping or ablation catheter (Fig. 9.13).

Favorable ablation sites usually have a pre potential or EGM onset of 35 msec or greater ahead of the surface QRS complex. When mapping within the RVOT, without particularly favorable activation mapping consideration of LV mapping should be undertaken prior to ablating. Pace mapping with software guided matching can be used to successfully locate infrequent PVC's within the EP lab (albeit with a somewhat lower success rate) and/or confirm the best site identified via activation mapping.

Electrophysiologic Study and Ablation of Idiopathic LVVT's

Idiopathic reentrant LVVT's make up less than 5% of the LVVT's encountered in general electrophysiologic practice (with the majority being ischemic, non-ischemic, outflow tract or high volume PVC's). However, their behavior and treatment differ such that they are deserving of special interest. With the electrocardiographic characteristics discussed previously, it is important to have a high index of suspicion dependent upon the resting and tachycardia ECG going into the invasive electrophysiologic study. During EP study it is important to induce the VT with a morphology that is consistent with the clinical VT. Entrainment from the inferoposterior septum of the left ventricle generally provides a favorable PPI-TCL with entrainment from the atrium remaining possible but usually showing a less favorable PPI-TCL.

Ablation of this rhythm is usually accomplished through targeting of purkinje potentials along the distal LV apex via a retroaortic (or transseptal) approach. Purkinje potentials are sharp high voltage fragmented signals distal to the LBBB. Radiofrequency energy applied at this point with an ablation catheter often would terminate the tachycardia and render the VT noninducible. With a loss of tachycardia inducibility the procedure is terminated and deemed successful.

VT of Special Consideration, Bundle Branch Reentry

Bundle branch reentry VT is a rare but important subtype of VT. These are mostly observed in patients with dilated cardiomyopathy with underlying conduction disease. When suspicious of BBR VT it is important to remember that BBRVT typically uses the diseased bundle branch (present on the resting 12 lead ECG and typically the left bundle branch) as the antegrade conducting limb of the circuit with the healthy limb as the retrograde limb. An important clue to bundle branch reentry if VT is presentation of tachycardia that displays the same QRS morphology at baseline but with findings of atrio-ventricular dissociation (Figs. 9.14 and 9.15).

Entrainment from the right ventricular apex usually results in a favorable PPI when compared to the tachycardia cycle length. It is

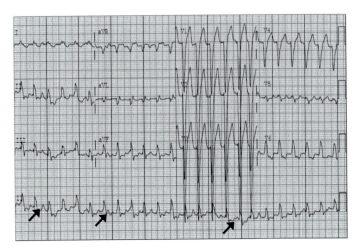

Fig. 9.14 Twelve lead ECG of a patient with Bundle Branch Reentry VT. The arrows denote p waves with dissociation of atrial (p waves) and ventricular (QRS) signals

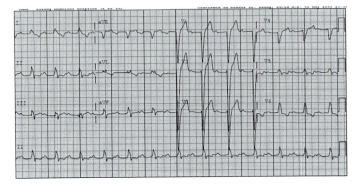

Fig. 9.15 Baseline 12 lead ECG of the same patient with bundle branch reentry VT during sinus rhythm. Note with exact same QRS morphology in sinus rhythm as during VT

usually possible to entrain the arrhythmia from the atrium given the necessary participation of the His-purkinje system in the tachycardia but with a long PPI relative to the tachycardia cycle length. As atrial activation is usually retrograde and thus dependent upon the reentrant circuit distal to the His bundle, changes in atrial cycle length are preceded by changes in the ventricular tachycardia cycle length. BBRVT typically has a morphology consistent with a full bundle branch block either left or more commonly right bundle branch block.

The ablation of this arrhythmia generally surrounds targeting the involved bundle branch with an ablation catheter, often during the induced ventricular tachycardia. Termination of the VT to sinus rhythm and loss of inducibility are appropriate endpoints for deeming the procedure successful and result in its termination. The right bundle potential is usually found apically to the His bundle on the septum. If the ablation catheter is positioned appropriately the right bundle potential can be separated from the His signal with a slight additional apical extension required to safely ablate the bundle branch and avoid the His bundle.

Ventricular Fibrillation Ablation

Ventricular fibrillation (VF) is a malignant arrhythmia responsible for sudden cardiac death. ICDs and medications including antiarrhythmics remain the standard of care for treatment of VF. However, the role of catheter ablation for the treatment of VF continues to evolve. Approaches to catheter ablation are based on the underlying conditions and substrate that trigger VF including idiopathic VF, Brugada syndrome, early repolarization syndrome, channelopathies, ischemia, or structural heart disease. Current approaches include mapping the site of the most frequent ventricular ectopy that has been identified on cardiac monitoring leading to VF. Majority of these PVCs that trigger VF arise from the Purkinje system, which makes an ideal target for catheter ablation [18]. Small studies and case series have demonstrated acute and long term effectiveness of catheter ablation of VF in select patient populations. One of the largest studies conducted to date was a prospective, multicenter study evaluating the efficacy of catheter ablation for VF storm after a myocardial infarction [19]. 110 patients with VF storm after an MI and without evidence of monomorphic VT underwent catheter ablation. The target ablation sites were Purkinje related ventricular ectopy triggering VF. The study demonstrated both short and long term suppression of recurrent VF storm. Thus, catheter ablation can be considered among patients with multiple episodes of VF despite maximally tolerated medical management.

Mapping Considerations

When mapping idiopathic VT in 3D, most commonly the window of interest will be set to capture the PVCs that spontaneously occur throughout the procedure. In some rare instances in which the patient can hemodynamically tolerate the VT, a faster map can be acquired. Most of the time, however, a map will be constructed that acquires electroanatomic (EA) data only on the spontaneous PVC locations.

Anatomy is always a concern when mapping PVCs, especially in the outflow tracts, due to the way the ventricle contracts on a PVC. Continuous acquisition of anatomy during normal sinus rhythm (NSR) can confuse the picture while mapping. While it is a slower process, it may be better to take a traditional "point by point" map on the 3D mapping system. This way, the entire map is built as a PVC map, rather than as a mix of NSR and PVCs. Another way to acquire a consistent anatomy is to use the CartoSound mapping technology. Each contour can be taken only on PVCs, so that a quick PVC-only anatomy can be built; EA data can then be plotted on the CartoSound map.

The key to setting a window of interest and mapping is to make sure only ventricular activation is being annotated. Points acquired by the tricuspid or mitral valve will have both atrial and ventricular signals. It is also important to be certain the points acquired are all in the intrinsic PVC, and not on a catheter-induced or clinically irrelevant PVC. This can become complicated when a patient presents with multiple morphologies of their PVC. It is usually best to try to map one PVC at a time, rather than constantly toggling between maps and risking missing beats. Parallel mapping now exists on one of the mapping systems (Biosense Webster's Carto system) which allows to map multiple PVC's simultaneously.

Another difficulty with mapping and treating PVC's is frequency on the day of procedure. A wide variety of factors, including strength of sedation, can play a role in how many PVC's a patient has during a procedure. Electrophysiologists are often frustrated to see a large PVC burden on a holter monitor, only to have the PVC's go silent or occur only rarely during a procedure. In these instances, pace-mapping is often performed, with varying results. In the past, this was difficult to map and very time-consuming. Because the matching of a paced morphology to the intrinsic PVC is subjective, the best the operator and EA mapper could do previously was to determine the best matches (usually placed on a scale with the 12 leads, e.g., "This is an 11/12 match") and mark these spots anatomically on the 3D map.

However, 3D mapping technology has advanced to make this process faster and more accurate. Software is now available on various mapping systems which allows the user to store the intrinsic PVC, or store multiple intrinsic PVCs, and then automatically tags and colors the map based on a percentage match to the various intrinsic PVCs (e.g., "This is a 98% match to the intrinsic PVC). This allows the electrophysiologist to pace-map multiple morphologies at a time (Fig. 9.16).

Mapping ischemic/non-ischemic VT has its own unique challenges. Like with idiopathic VT, it is rare to map activation during VT, due to hemodynamic instability. Because VT that comes from these patients is usually reentrant, in the rare case that EA mapping is performed, the window of interest should be set at 90% of the cycle length, with a distinct, sharp peak of a body surface ECG lead as the "time zero" reference point.

Usually, however, substrate mapping will be performed. Setting the window of interest for mapping ischemic/non-ischemic substrate is not complicated, but it is critical to get it right. Rather than collecting timing, the map will collect and represent bipolar voltage. Usually a scale of 0.5–1.5 mv is set – this makes every-

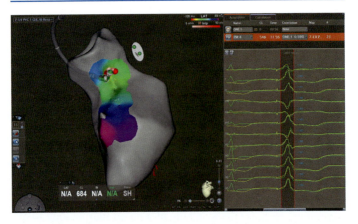

Fig. 9.16 Paso Technology (Biosense Webster, Diamond Bar, CA). Pace-match of 98% was obtained at the at earliest site of activation of an LVOT PVC. Ablation strategy is targeted toward highest percentage pace map matches when intrinsic PVCs occur rarely

thing below 0.5 mv to be considered dense scar, and everything above 1.5 mv to be considered healthy tissue. Everything between 0.5 and 1.5 mv is then displayed on a color scale representing various levels of tissue health. This color scale between 0.5 and 1.5 mv will usually show up on the "border zone" of dense scar. With a high density map, electrophysiologists will also be able to find channels of viable tissue through the dense scar, which helps locate the zones of slow conduction through the scar responsible for the reentrant tachycardias. Close attention should be paid to fragmented electrograms and mid-diastolic potentials, as these also represent zones of slow conduction through scar areas. Paso pace-map matching software can also be used to identify the critical isthmus for ischemic VT. If the VT is induced or observed during the procedure, the morphology can be saved in Paso, and pacing can be performed through scar areas to identify VT match (Figs. 9.17 and 9.18).

Substrate mapping can be problematic when careful attention is not applied to the acquired points. The points should be consistent. Mapping in SR is preferable, but not always possible. When

9 Ventricular Tachyarrhythmias

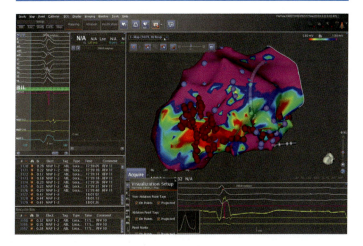

Fig. 9.17 3D substrate map of ischemic VT. Red areas are dense scar (<0.5mv). Purple areas are healthy tissue (>0.5 mv). Yellow, green and blue represent damaged "border zone" tissue. Ablation strategy here targeted a critical isthmus through the middle of the scar

mapping in SR, the 3D mapper must be careful only to take sinus points; paced beats or catheter-induced PVC's should be discarded. When mapping a paced ventricle, the window of interest must be set to exclude the pacing spike which will be present on the mapping catheter. If the window does not exclude this pacing spike, the map will confuse it with an actual electrogram. The most important, basic rule while mapping a substrate: anything inside the window is "seen" and measured as voltage by the mapping system! Be sure to exclude anything that is not intrinsic EGM.

A final difficulty to overcome when substrate mapping is the anatomical challenge of the left ventricle. Large papillary muscles, chordae tendonae, and trabeculation are all anatomical challenges that make catheter maneuvering and mapping difficult. For this reason, phased array ICE is often used. When paired with CartoSound technology, the 3D map can actually display internal structures like papillary muscles, giving important knowledge for how to navigate and where to map (Fig. 9.19).

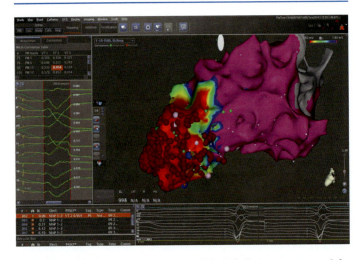

Fig. 9.18 Paso technology in ischemic VT. Apical scar was targeted for extensive ablation. Paso revealed two channels (small red dots inside of dark blue tags), representing 95% matches to two different VT morphologies. These VTs were non-inducible post-ablation

Additionally, with these internal structures, it can be hard to know whether or not the catheter is in good contact with the tissue. If the catheter does not have good contact, and a point is acquired, the map will read the lack of electrogram as dense scar. This can be misleading, plotting scar on the 3D map while the catheter is actually floating off the tissue. Contact force sensing technology can solve this problem. By measuring the actual contact and force of contact against the tissue, operators can know whether they are in contact with the tissue and apply consistent force of contact throughout the map. The confusion surrounding "internal" versus "real" points on a map is virtually eliminated with a contact force sensing catheter.

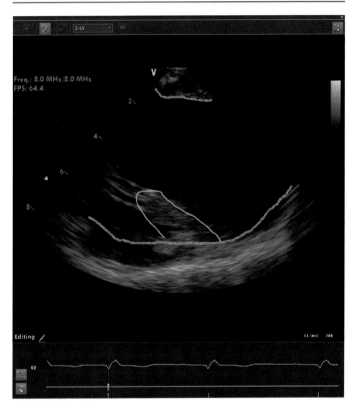

Fig. 9.19 Papillary muscle drawn on the CartoSound technology. Papillary muscles are then represented in 3D on the map, so the catheter navigation and contact assessment can take these into account

Noninvasive Radiation Therapy for Ventricular Tachycardia

Catheter ablation of ventricular arrhythmias can be effective in select patients. However, procedural success can be limited due to inability to target ablation site with catheters due to challenging anatomies, and other factors and the procedure may also be too high risk for some patients. Patients who cannot undergo invasive procedures or those have failed multiple ablations are left with very limited treatment options. Stereotactic body radiation therapy (SBRT) has emerged as a palliative option for refractory ventricular arrhythmias. SBRT utilizes non-invasive electrophysiology mapping to identify scar or arrhythmic substrate and delivers targeted high dose radiation (25 Gy in a single fraction). Cuculich et al. recently reported longer-term results from SBRT performed in 19 patients with either treatment-refractory VT or PVC-related cardiomyopathy. The median follow-up was 34 months (7.9–60.1 months). Overall survival at 1, 2, and 3 years was 74%, 53%, and 46%, respectively. Nine deaths occurred, with 4 possibly related to the treatment. Late serious adverse events (>6 months) were rare [20]. The use of SBRT for patients with refractory ventricular arrhythmias is increasing, but ongoing translational science work and clinical trials will be needed to address many outstanding questions regarding this new therapy for ventricular arrhythmias.

Summary

Ventricular tachyarrhythmias are an increasingly common occurrence with the growing ICD population. Knowledge of the electrophysiologic characteristics and treatment of these arrhythmias continues to grow. For the majority of these patients recurrences downstream are a constant risk and may require ongoing antiarrhythmic drug therapy for complete suppression. In experienced hands it is possible to study and treat these arrhythmias successfully in a safe fashion. However, as our knowledge of the benefit of VT ablation grows it is becoming increasingly clear that this procedure, when performed properly, can further reduce the risk of subsequent ICD shocks and mortality [21, 22].

References

1. Farzaneh-Far A, Lerman BB. Idiopathic ventricular outflow tract tachycardia. Heart. 2005;91:136–8.
2. Brugada P, Brugada J, Mont L, Smeets J, Andries EW. A new approach to the differential diagnosis of a regular tachycardia with a wide QRS complex. Circulation. 1991;83:1649–59.

3. Vereckei A, Duray G, Szénási G, Altemose GT, Miller JM. New algorithm using only lead aVR for differential diagnosis of wide QRS complex tachycardia. Heart Rhythm. 2008;5:89–98.
4. Pava LF, Perafán P, Badiel M, et al. R-wave peak time at DII: a new criterion for differentiating between wide complex QRS tachycardias. Heart Rhythm. 2010;7:922–6.
5. Daniels DV, Lu YY, Morton JB, et al. Idiopathic epicardial left ventricular tachycardia originating remote from the sinus of Valsalva: electrophysiological characteristics, catheter ablation, and identification from the 12-lead electrocardiogram. Circulation. 2006;113:1659–66.
6. Betensky BP, Park RE, Marchlinski FE, et al. The V(2) transition ratio: a new electrocardiographic criterion for distinguishing left from right ventricular outflow tract tachycardia origin. J Am Coll Cardiol. 2011;57:2255–62.
7. Efremidis M, Vlachos K, Kyriakopoulou M, et al. The RV(1)-V(3) transition ratio: a novel electrocardiographic criterion for the differentiation of right versus left outflow tract premature ventricular complexes. Heart Rhythm O2. 2021;2:521–8.
8. Stevenson WG, Friedman PL, Sager PT, et al. Exploring postinfarction reentrant ventricular tachycardia with entrainment mapping. J Am Coll Cardiol. 1997;29:1180–9.
9. De Maria E, Giacopelli D, Borghi A, Modonesi L, Cappelli S. Antitachycardia pacing programming in implantable cardioverter defibrillator: a systematic review. World J Cardiol. 2017;9:429–36.
10. Cantillon DJ, Wilkoff BL. Antitachycardia pacing for reduction of implantable cardioverter-defibrillator shocks. Heart Rhythm. 2015;12:1370–5.
11. Sesselberg HW, Moss AJ, McNitt S, et al. Ventricular arrhythmia storms in postinfarction patients with implantable defibrillators for primary prevention indications: a MADIT-II substudy. Heart Rhythm. 2007;4:1395–402.
12. Vaseghi M, Gima J, Kanaan C, et al. Cardiac sympathetic denervation in patients with refractory ventricular arrhythmias or electrical storm: intermediate and long-term follow-up. Heart Rhythm. 2014;11:360–6.
13. Cronin EM, Bogun FM, Maury P, et al. 2019 HRS/EHRA/APHRS/LAHRS expert consensus statement on catheter ablation of ventricular arrhythmias. Europace. 2019;21:1143–4.
14. Yamashita S, Sacher F, Mahida S, et al. Image integration to guide catheter ablation in scar-related ventricular tachycardia. J Cardiovasc Electrophysiol. 2016;27:699–708.
15. Bhakta D, Miller JM. Principles of electroanatomic mapping. Indian Pacing Electrophysiol J. 2008;8:32–50.
16. Aziz Z, Shatz D, Raiman M, et al. Targeted ablation of ventricular tachycardia guided by wavefront discontinuities during sinus rhythm: a new functional substrate mapping strategy. Circulation. 2019;140:1383–97.

17. Sánchez-Quintana D, Ho SY, Climent V, Murillo M, Cabrera JA. Anatomic evaluation of the left phrenic nerve relevant to epicardial and endocardial catheter ablation: implications for phrenic nerve injury. Heart Rhythm. 2009;6:764–8.
18. Anderson RD, Kumar S, Kalman JM, et al. Catheter ablation of ventricular fibrillation. Heart Lung Circ. 2019;28:110–22.
19. Komatsu Y, Hocini M, Nogami A, et al. Catheter ablation of refractory ventricular fibrillation storm after myocardial infarction. Circulation. 2019;139:2315–25.
20. Cuculich P. Longer Term Results From A Phase I/II Study Of EP-guided Noninvasive Cardiac Radioablation For Treatment Of Ventricular Tachycardia (ENCORE-VT). Heart Rhythm Society 2020 virtual meeting, 2020.
21. Reddy VY, Reynolds MR, Neuzil P, et al. Prophylactic catheter ablation for the prevention of defibrillator therapy. N Engl J Med. 2007;357:2657–65.
22. Kuck KH, Schaumann A, Eckardt L, et al. Catheter ablation of stable ventricular tachycardia before defibrillator implantation in patients with coronary heart disease (VTACH): a multicentre randomised controlled trial. Lancet. 2010;375:31–40.

Hereditary Arrhythmias

10

Ido Goldenberg, Alon Barsheshet, and David T. Huang

Abstract

Ventricular tachyarrhythmias (ventricular tachycardia [VT] or ventricular fibrillation [VF]) are associated with syncope, aborted cardiac arrest (ACA) or sudden cardiac death (SCD). Patients will experience syncope, ACA, or SCD depending on the duration of the VT and whether VT degenerates into VF.

The etiology of these life-threatening hereditary arrhythmias can be classified according to whether structural heart disease is present or not. Structural causes of hereditary arrhythmias include hypertrophic cardiomyopathy (HCM), and arrhythmogenic right ventricular cardiomyopathy/dysplasia (ARVC/D). Most of the nonstructural causes of hereditary

---

I. Goldenberg
Rochester General Hospital, Rochester, NY, USA

University of Rochester Medical Center, Rochester, NY, USA

A. Barsheshet
The Rabin Medical Center, Tel-Aviv University, Tel-Aviv, Israel

D. T. Huang (✉)
University of Rochester Medical Center, Rochester, NY, USA
e-mail: david_huang@urmc.rochester.edu

© The Author(s), under exclusive license to Springer Nature Switzerland AG 2023
D. T. Huang et al. (eds.), *Cardiac Electrophysiology in Clinical Practice*, In Clinical Practice,
https://doi.org/10.1007/978-3-031-41479-4_10

arrhythmias are cardiac channelopathies (disorders involving mutations in genes encoding cardiac ion channels) that include the congenital long QT syndromes (LQTS), Brugada syndrome, and catecholaminergic polymorphic ventricular tachycardia (CPVT). Inherited infiltrative cardiomyopathies, such as Fabry disease, are also an important cause of arrhythmias.

This chapter will focus on the clinical and genetic aspects of the LQTS, Brugada syndrome, and ARVC/D, CPVT. It should be noted that these genetic syndromes exhibit incomplete penetrance (i.e., the likelihood that a disease-causing mutation will have a phenotypic expression in a mutation-positive subject) and variable expressivity (i.e., different level of phenotypic expression), implicating environmental factors and possibly other genetic modifiers in the etiology of these diseases.

Keywords

Hereditary arrhythmias · Ventricular tachycardia · Long QT syndrome · Brugada · Torsades de pointes · ARVC/D · Cardiac devices therapy · Fabry disease

Long QT Syndrome

Introduction

The long QT syndrome (LQTS) is a hereditary arrhythmia syndrome characterized by structurally normal heart and delayed ventricular repolarization manifested on the ECG as abnormal QT interval prolongation and T wave abnormalities.

LQTS is commonly associated with syncope, however SCD can occur due to torsade de pointes. This is a form of polymorphic ventricular tachycardia that is associated with a prolonged QT interval preceding the arrhythmia. The estimated prevalence of LQTS is 1:2000–2500 of apparently healthy live-births [1]. About 85% of the reported cases are inherited from one of the parents, with the remaining 15% of affected patients having de novo mutations. There is a slight female predominance that is more prominent after puberty.

The first descriptions identified two patterns of inheritance: autosomal dominant and autosomal recessive. The most common form is the autosomal dominant form, also called Romano-Ward syndrome. The autosomal recessive form, also called Jervell-Lange-Nielsen syndrome, is a severe form of LQTS associated with congenital deafness.

To date, over 600 mutations have been recognized in 13 LQTS genes. Three main genes associated with LQT1, LQT2 and LQT3, respectively account for 90% of genotype-positive LQTS patients and about 75% of all patients with LQTS [2].

Importantly, about 40% of patients with genotype-positive LQTS may have a baseline QRS that is within normal range [3].

The LQTS is a leading cause of SCD in young patients with a structurally normal heart. Without treatment, the mortality rate can reach 21% within 1 year of the first episode of syncope [4].

Mechanism of LQTS

The molecular mechanisms in LQTS can be associated with genetic defects that lead to a decrease in repolarizing potassium currents or increased depolarizing sodium and calcium channels. These genes mutations lead to abnormal ion channels associated with prolongation of the myocardial action potential. The prolonged action potential may be explained by at least two mechanisms: (1) it increases the calcium current available sodium channel reactivation during the repolarizing phase which leads to the development of early afterdepolarizations and subsequent triggered activity. (2) it preferentially occurs in the epicardium compared to the endocardium, resulting in an increase in transmural dispersion of repolarization which in turn, increases the probability of reentrant arrhythmias [4].

A. LQT1

This clinical syndrome is caused by loss of function (LOF) mutations in KCNQ1, encoding the alpha-subunit of the slowly activating potassium channel. This leads to reduced current of the slow component of the delayed rectifier IK current, the most significant determinant of the cardiac action potential. In fact most cases of AR JLN Syndrome are caused by either heterozygous or homozygous mutations in KCNQ1.

B. LQT2

LQT2 is associated with LOF mutations in KCNH2 (Herg), ultimately leading to reduced rapidly activating potassium current.

C. LQT3

This is associated with gain of function mutations in SCN5A which results in increased sodium current during the plateau and the late phase of the action potential.

D. LQT 4–16

13 genes, in addition to the ones described above, that were identified account for 5% of clinically diagnosed LQTS. The mechanism of action of each of these mutations is beyond the scope of this chapter.

Diagnosis and Classification

The diagnosis of LQTS is based on measurement of the corrected QT (QTc) on the ECG, clinical history, and/or genetic testing. A recent expert consensus statement [3] suggested that a diagnosis of LQTS can be made if one or more of the following criteria are fulfilled: (1) In the presence of a very prolonged QTc ($\geq$500 ms) in repeated 12- lead ECG and in the absence of a secondary cause for QT prolongation; (2) If a prolonged QTc is identified after a syncopal event in the absence of acquired causes of QT prolongation; (3) In the presence of an LQTS risk score (the Schwartz-Moss risk score based on personal and family history, symptomatology, and ECG) [5] $\geq$3.5; (4) In the presence of a pathogenic mutation in one of the LQTS genes.

It should be noted that about 25% of patients with genetically confirmed LQTS exhibit QTc within normal range [6]. Four major provocative tests have been proposed to unmask LQTS patients with normal range QT at rest: (1) change from a supine to standing position [7], (2) during the recovery phase of exercise testing [8], (3) infusion of epinephrine [9], or (4) Adenosine-induced, sudden bradycardia and subsequent tachycardia [10].

LQTS is classified into 13 types according to the identified 13 LQTS associated genes with LQTS types 1–3 being the most common types of LQTS. LQTS type 1 accounts for 30–35% of cases of LQTS and involves a loss of function mutation in the alpha subunit of the slow delayed rectifier potassium channel KCNQ1; the current through this channel is known as I_{Ks}.

LQTS type 2 accounts for 25–30% of cases of LQTS and involves loss of function mutations in the alpha subunit of the rapid delayed rectifier potassium channel KCNH2 (or hERG); the current through this channel is known as I_{Kr}.

LQTS type 3 accounts for 5–10% of cases of LQTS and involves a gain of function mutation in the alpha subunit of the sodium channel SCN5A, the current through this channel is known as I_{Na}.

LQTS types 4 through 14 are rare, each type accounts for less than 1% of cases of LQTS. LQT5 involves a mutation in the beta subunit KCNE1 (or MinK) which co-assembles with KCNQ1. LQT6 involves a mutation in the beta subunit KCNE2 (or MiRP1) which co-assembles with KCNH2. LQT7 involves a mutation in the potassium channel gene KCNJ2; the current through this channel is called I_{K1}. It leads to Andersen-Tawil syndrome, which is associated with periodic paralysis and physical abnormalities including short stature, micrognathia, dental abnormalities, low-set ears, widely spaced eyes, and unusual curving of the fingers or toes (clinodactyly). LQT8 involves a mutation in the L type calcium channel encoded by the gene CACNA1c. It leads to Timothy's syndrome, which is associated with a very poor prognosis and also fusion of the fingers or toes (syndactyly), flattened nose, small teeth, autism, and possible cardiac structural anomalies.

Genetic testing may have an important role in the diagnosis, risk stratification, and management of carriers of LQTS mutations. Currently, genetic testing is usually performed when there is a clinical suspicion of LQTS and for confirmatory testing among family members of identified probands.

Risk Stratification

Genotype-Phenotype Correlation

Genotype-phenotype correlation in the LQTS has been the most active line of research among the structurally normal heart diseases. It has been recognized that there is an association between the genetic background and clinical characteristics of the LQTS including electrocardiographic features, triggers for cardiac events, risk stratification and prognosis.

Moss et al. [11] have demonstrated that the ST-T wave repolarization pattern on the ECG differs among the three common LQTS genotypes. Patients with LQT1 typically have a broad-based T-wave pattern; patients with LQT2 exhibit a low amplitude bifid T-wave, whereas in LQT3, T-wave is usually peaked and late onset.

Importantly, cardiac events in LQTS were shown to be associated with gene-specific triggers. Patients with the LQT1 genotype are at a higher risk for arrhythmic events triggered by sympathetic activation induced by exercise. Among the different types of exercise, swimming was shown to be a specific trigger for LQT1 patients [12, 13]. Patients with the LQT2 genotype are at a higher risk for arrhythmic events triggered by emotional stress, including anger, fear, startle, or sudden noise during sleep. Patients with the LQT3 genotype experience arrhythmic events mostly during sleep or at rest without emotional arousal.

Risk stratification among non-genotyped LQTS patients relies on a combined assessment of clinical and ECG factors. Figure 10.1 shows a suggested risk stratification scheme for non-genotyped patients with LQTS. Patients may be classified into three main risk categories: (1) The very high-risk group includes patients with a history of ACA and/or spontaneous Torsades de pointes; these patients require an implantable cardioverter defibrillator (ICD) implantation for secondary prevention of SCD; (2) The high-risk group includes subjects with history of prior syncope or QTc > 500 ms, and (3) the low risk group includes those with QTc duration of ≤500 ms without prior syncope event [2].

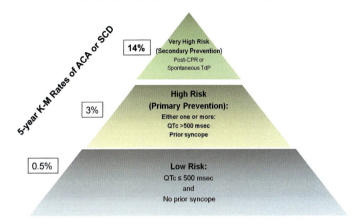

Fig. 10.1 5-year K-M Rates of ACA or SCD

Risk stratification among genotyped LQTS patients can be based on genotype-specific factors found to affect the phenotypic expression in patients with LQTS; those risk factors include age, gender, the post partum time period, menopause, prior syncope, mutation location, type of mutation (missense/ non-missense), the biophysical function of the mutation and response to betablockers [14, 15]. Figs. 10.2 and 10.3 show suggested risk stratification schemes for patients with LQT1 and LQT2, respectively.

The rare forms of LQTS Jervell-Lange-Nielsen syndrome (autosomal recessive inheritance form of LQTS) and Andersen-Tawil syndrome (LQTS type 7) are both associated with very poor prognoses (unless ICD is implanted); Patients with these syndromes experience life threatening arrhythmic events at an early age. Similarly, patients with multiple LQTS-associated mutations, particularly double mutations affecting the same gene, have been associated with a greater risk for life threatening arrhythmic events than patients who harbor a single mutation [16].

Gender and Risk of Arrhythmias

As mentioned above, there is a slight female predominance in patients with LQTS. Additionally, among patients already diagnosed with LQTS, prior studies have shown that there is an

a Rate of ACA/SCD in LQT1 Females by Mutation-Location

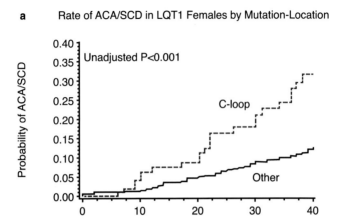

b Rate of ACA/SCD in LQT1 Females by Mutation-Location

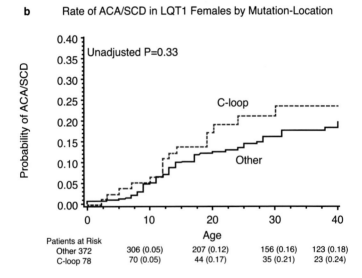

Fig. 10.2 Kaplan-Meier estimates of the cumulative probability of aborted cardiac arrest or sudden cardiac death in (**a**) women with LQT1 and (**b**) men with LQT1, by mutation location. ACA = aborted cardiac arrest; C-loop mutations = cytoplasmic-loop mutations; LQT1 = long QT syndrome type 1; SCD = sudden cardiac death

10 Hereditary Arrhythmias

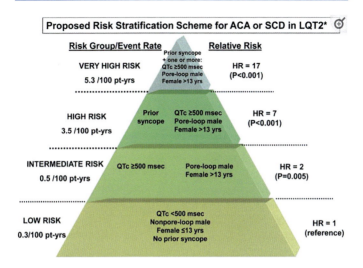

Fig. 10.3 Peroposed Risk Stratification Scheme for ACA or SCD in LQT2*

increased risk of cardiovascular events (CEs) after the onset of adolescence, and during the perimenopause period. The increase in the risk of the perimenopause period was shown to be more pronounced in women with LQTS2 genetic mutation [17].

In contrast, the risk of CEs in men is attenuated after the onset of adolescence. The mechanisms leading to the different risk between men and women has been attributed to the modulating effects on the potassium channels associated with the cardiac action potential.

Estrogen and progesterone were shown to have varying effects on IKs and IKr currents. Testosterone, on the other hand increases potassium channel currents, resulting in a shorter corrected QT (QTc) in both animal and human studies.

More recently, the use of oral contraceptives was studied with relation to the risk of CEs in female patients with LQTS. It was found that progestin-only OC therapy is associated with increased risk of CEs in women with congenital LQTS [18]. Concomitantly beta-blocker therapy significantly attenuates the risk of CEs during progestin-only OC use. Importantly, the risk associated with OC use is more pronounced in females with LQT2 gene mutations.

Management

In general, the treatment of LQTS consists of lifestyle modifications, medical therapy with beta-blockers, ICD and/or surgical therapy. The ACC/AHA/ESC guidelines [19] and a recently published expert consensus statement [3] recommend lifestyle modifications for all patients with a diagnosis of LQTS. Beta-blockers are recommended as a Class I indication for all patients with a clinical diagnosis of LQTS and as a Class IIa indication for patients with a genetic diagnosis of LQTS who have a normal QTc duration. Although there are limited data on the most effective dosage of beta-blockers, full dosing adjusted for age and weight is recommended. Abrupt discontinuation of beta-blockers should be avoided as this may cause exacerbation [3]. Implantation of an ICD is recommended for LQTS patients who experience an aborted cardiac arrest (class I indication) or for patients who had syncope and/or VT despite beta-blockers therapy (class IIa indication). The recently published expert consensus statement [3] recommends performing left cardiac sympathetic denervation (LCSD) in high-risk patients with a diagnosis of LQTS in whom ICD therapy is contraindicated or refused and/or beta-blockers are either not effective in preventing syncope/arrhythmias, not tolerated, or contraindicated (class IIa indication). In addition, the consensus statement has added that sodium channel blockers can be useful, as add-on therapy, for LQT3 patients with a QTc >500 ms who shorten their QTc by >40 ms following an acute oral sodium channel blocker test (class IIa indication) [3].

Lifestyle Modifications

The fact that patients with certain genotypes are more likely to experience their events under well-defined circumstances may provide insights into preventive measures. Patients with LQT1 have most of their events during exercise. Therefore, they should avoid strenuous exercise activity (particularly swimming) without supervision, and those at intermediate or high risk should not engage into competitive sports [3, 19]. Patients with LQT2 should be advised to avoid unexpected auditory stimuli as their cardiac events are predominantly associated with sudden arousal [17, 20]. Removal of loud noise stimuli at home and work such as elimination of alarm clocks, door bells and telephone ringing is usually recommended. LQT3 patients mainly experience events during sleep and at rest, and should be considered for a special intercom system in the bedroom. All patients with LQTS should avoid drugs known to prolong QT interval, or affect potassium and magnesium level. It is important to Identify and correct electrolyte abnormalities that may occur during diarrhea, vomiting, metabolic conditions, or imbalanced diets for weight loss [3].

Beta-Blockers

Beta-blocker therapy is the mainstay treatment of patients with LQTS. The efficacy of this therapy in LQTS has been demonstrated in multiple studies. Moss et al. [21] have reported the efficacy of beta-blockers in 869 LQTS patients. Beta-blocker therapy was associated with a significant reduction in the rate of cardiac events in probands (0.97 ± 1.42 to 0.31 ± 0.86 events per year, $p < 0.001$) and in affected family members (0.26 ± 0.84 to 0.15 ± 0.69 events per year, $p < 0.001$). In another study among 549 LQT1 and 422 LQT2 patients from the International LQTS Registry, we have found that Beta-blocker therapy was associated with a prominent risk-reduction in high-risk patients, including a 67% reduction ($p = 0.02$) in LQT1 males and a 71% reduction ($p < 0.001$) in LQT2 females [22].

The protective effects of beta-blockers among LQTS patients may also depend on mutation location. We have shown among 860 patients with genetically confirmed LQT1 that beta-blocker therapy was associated with a significant 88% reduction in the risk of life-threatening cardiac events among LQT1 carriers of the cytoplasmic loops (C-loop) missense mutations ($p = 0.02$), whereas among LQT1 carriers of non-C-loop missense mutations there was no significant reduction in the risk for life threatening cardiac events (HR 0.82, $p = 0.68$) [23]. It is known that the C-loops play an important role in the sympathetic regulation of the KCNQ1 channel [24]. Cellular expression studies have suggested that there is a combination of decrease in basal function and altered adrenergic regulation of the I_{Ks} channel in patients with C-loops missense mutations that may provide a potential explanation why beta-blockers are particularly effective in patients with this type of mutation [23].

The benefit associated with the various beta-blocker subtypes in the management of LQTS may not be equal. Two studies [22, 25] may suggest that metoprolol is less effective than Atenolol, Nadolol or Propranolol among LQT1 and LQT2 patients. Evidence suggests that treatment with nadolol results in the greatest risk reduction in the overall LQTS population, proven to be effective mainly in LQT1 and LQT2 [2].

The clinical effect of the beta-blocker type may not be causally related to its specific effect on the QTc interval. For example, propranolol may offer greater reductions in the QTc interval, but it is suggested that its efficacy is mainly in patients with LQT1 [2].

Adherence to beta-blocker therapy is of utmost importance and all patients must be counseled on it. A recent real-world study regarding pharmacy dispensing data in patients with LQTS found that over 50% of patients had suboptimal adherence to the prescribed beta-blocker therapy. Therefore, the risk reduction associated with optimal beta-blocker therapy adherence and dosing may be much greater than what is reported.

Assessing sufficient beta-blocker effect during therapy can be done with the demonstration of blunting of heart rate response with exercise testing. The aim should not be for QTc shortening, but a decrement of 15–20% during maximum exercise to demonstrate adequate effect and adherence.

Adjunctive Medical Therapies

Mexiletine has been demonstrated to be efficacious in addition to beta-blockers in the treatment of patients with LQTS. In fact, patients with LQT3, who have a gain of function variant in there

Nav1.5 sodium channel, mexiletine therapy resulted in a 60 ms reduction in QTc interval and reducing CEs. A small study showed that adjunctive therapy with mexiletine to beta blockers may provide added therapeutic efficacy [2].

Other medications that have been used in small studies include nicorandil and ranolazine through their effects on potentiation of potassium channels and blockade of sodium channels, respectively. However, these therapies require further validation in future large-scale clinical trials.

Potassium Supplementation

Potassium supplementation and spironolactone were proposed for patients with LQT2 who exhibit mutation of the KCNH2 gene. KCNH2 function is highly dependent on the extracellular potassium. It has been suggested that potassium administration will increase serum potassium level and improve repolarization abnormalities. Two small studies have shown that potassium supplements and spironolactone are associated with a significant shortening of the QTc [26, 27]. Unfortunately, there are no data that potassium supplements or spironolactone can decrease the risk of cardiac events.

Sodium Channel Blockers

Over the last decade, sodium channel blockers such as mexiletine and flecainide have been investigated as a potential treatment option for patients with LQT3. Both Mexilitine [4] and Flecainide [28–32] administration are associated with significant shortening of the QT interval among LQT3 patients.

Treatment Considerations During Pregnancy

Each stage of pregnancy poses a different risk in specific LQTS population and understanding those risks as well as the safety of treatment options is paramount to care for these patients. For example, hyperemesis can be associated with the first trimester. In severe cases, this leads to poor absorption of medications and also hypokalemia and hypomagnesemia. These women should be monitored more closely with supplementations provided. It should be noted that almost all antiemetic medications are QT prolonging and should be avoided is possible. If used, ECG monitoring with frequent electrolyte checks should be done until symptoms of hyperemesis subside [2, 33].

To date, continuation of beta-blockers is considered safe during pregnancy and reduces maternal risk especially in the postpartum period. It is important to explain that avoiding maternal arrhythmic complications increases the chance of a healthy fetus [33].

There is a broad safety data regarding propranolol during pregnancy given its pregnancy related hyperthyroidism indication and non-selective mechanism. However, high-risk LQTS patients usually may continue nadolol without significant issues.

In the largest study on pregnancy including patients with LQTS, the pregnancy period was associated with fewer events when compared to the pre-pregnancy period. The postpartum period is considered a proarrhythmic trigger in long QT syndrome, especially in type 2, which poses the greatest risk of arrhythmias. Importantly, the risk remains elevated for a minimum of 9 months postpartum especially for the type 2 patient population. During this postpartum period, propranolol is a god option as it can be taken while breastfeeding, while nadolol is generally not recommended but often continued if women have been stable on it during pregnancy [33].

Device Therapies

In patients with LQTS and a history of cardiac arrest, there is a clear indication for ICD insertion for secondary prevention. The decision for primary prevention ICD is more nuanced and should take into consideration the risk of sustaining a life-threatening ventricular tachyarrhythmia vs the risk of device related complications. These device related complications include inappropriate shocks, device infection, lead malfunction, and psychological consequences among others [2].

The intravenous dual-chamber ICD may be more advantageous than a subcutaneous ICD in LQTS patients for several reasons. First, there is more experience with the intravenous ICD among these patients. Second, the atrial overdrive pacing function may offer benefits for treatment of acute ventricular arrhythmias or for their prevention in pause dependent QT prolongation [2].

A pacemaker therapy without an ICD can be considered in certain patients including those with pause-dependent or bradycardia-related TdP as pacing may improve QT changes associated with heart rate variability. A pacemaker may also provide additional benefit in those patients not able to tolerate adequate doses of beta-blocker therapy [2].

Left Cardiac Sympathetic Denervation

This mode of therapy can reduce the number of CEs in patients who are already taking beta-blockers or in those who have failed beta-blocker therapy [2].

Technical Aspects

QTc Values The normal and prolonged QTc values depend on age and gender. Suggested QTc values for diagnosing QTc prolongation are: QTc >460 ms during childhood (ages 1–15 years), QTc >450 ms for adult males, and QTc >470 ms for adult females [32].

QT and QTc Measurement The QT interval should be determined as a mean value derived from at least 3–5 cardiac cycles, and is measured from the beginning of the QRS complex to the end of the T wave.

The QT measurement should be made in leads II and V5 or V6, with the longest value being used. The main difficulty lies when there are T and U waves that are close together. When T-wave deflections of a near-equal amplitude result in a biphasic T wave, the QT interval is measured to the time of final return to baseline. If a second low amplitude repolarization wave interrupts the terminal portion of the T wave, it is difficult to determine whether the second deflection is a biphasic T wave or an early-occurring U wave. In such cases, it is best to record both the QT (measured at the end of the first deflection) and the QTU (measured at the end of the second deflection) intervals [5].

The Bazett formula is widely used to correct the QT interval for heart rate (QTc); QTc equals QT divided by the square root of the R-R interval (all intervals should be measured in seconds).

Epinephrine QT Stress Test This provocative test may aid in unmasking individuals with concealed LQT1 [6]. There are two available protocols: by bolus infusion (Shimizu protocol) or an incremental, escalating infusion (Mayo protocol). According to the Mayo protocol, [6] after 10 min of rest, 12 lead ECG recording speed was set at 50 mm/s, baseline parameters were obtained (including QT and QTc), and then an infusion of epinephrine was initiated at 0.025 µg/kg/min. After 10 minutes of the infusion, the measurements were repeated. The epinephrine infusion was then increased sequentially to 0.05, and 0.1 µg/kg/min, and the measurements were repeated 5 minutes after each dose increase. The epinephrine infusion was then discontinued, and measurements were obtained 5 and 10 min afterwards. A paradoxical response characterized by uncorrected QT lengthening ($\Delta QT \geq 30$ ms) rather than expected shortening appears diagnostic for LQT1 (with a sensitivity and specificity of 92% and 86%, respectively).

Brugada Syndrome

Incidence and Etiology

Brugada syndrome is another familial disorder with structurally normal heart that involves mutations in genes encoding myocyte ion channels. Brugada syndrome is characterized by a specific ECG pattern of coved-type ST-segment elevation in the right precordial leads (V1 through V3) accompanied by a susceptibility to polymorphic VT and SCD [34]. Brugada syndrome prevalence has been estimated at 1 per 2000 people worldwide. The prevalence is higher in Asian and Southeast Asian countries, especially Thailand, Philippines and Japan [35, 36].

Brugada syndrome is typically inherited through an autosomal dominant mode of transmission. To date, 12 Brugada syndrome-associated genes have been reported [37], with all mutations leading to either a decrease in the inward sodium or calcium current or an increase in outward potassium current.

Approximately 25% of cases of Brugada syndrome result from mutations in the SCN5A gene that encodes for the α subunit of the cardiac sodium channel. Overall, the genetic cause has been identified for only 30% of clinically diagnosed Brugada syndrome patients.

Clinical Presentation

Overall there is a male predominance (about 90% of cases). The first symptoms typically occur in the third to fourth decade of life. These symptoms may range from syncope to SCD. That being said, the majority of newly diagnosed patients are asymptomatic (about 64%) or have a history of syncope (30%). Only about 6% of patients present with a cardiac arrest. Conditions that may bring about type-1 Brugada pattern include electrolyte imbalances, hyperthermia, fever, and sodium channel-blocking drugs [38].

Diagnosis

Three ECG patterns associated with Brugada syndrome were described.

Type 1 is characterized by a J point elevation ≥ 2 mm (0.2 mV), a coved ST-segment elevation followed by a negative T wave. This ECG pattern is diagnostic of Brugada syndrome. Type 2 has a J point elevation ≥ 2 mm, ST-segment elevation has a saddleback appearance, and then either a positive or biphasic T wave.

Type 3 has either a saddleback or coved appearance with a J point elevation <2 mm, and an ST-segment elevation of <1 mm.

Type 2 and type 3 ECG are not diagnostic of the Brugada syndrome.

The most recent expert consensus statement recommends the following criteria in diagnosing Brugada Syndrome:

1. A spontaneous type 1 (coved type) BrS-ECG as described above
2. Type 1 Brugada syndrome unmasked by sodium channel blockers or fever only when having a type 2 or type 3 ECG at baseline and when accompanied by at least one additional criterion from the 'Shanghai Score System'. This score system takes into account ECG patterns, clinical history, family history, and genetic testing in the prediction of a true Brugada Syndrome diagnosis.

It is important to exclude phenocopies which are other conditions that may explain a coved-type ECG. If the baseline ECG lacks the spontaneous type 1 Brugada pattern, then sodium channel blocker challenge should only be performed if the clinical suspicion remains high. This is because there is an estimated rate of 5% positive tests in healthy subjects and the consequences of treatment can be life-changing. These can include patients who have had a cardiac arrest or arrhythmias while febrile, patients with a family history of Brugada Syndrome, or unexplained SCD.

Genetics of Brugada Syndrome

Mutations in the SCN5A gene encoding the cardiac sodium channel have been identified in patients with Brugada Syndrome. These lead to a dysfunctional sodium channel at the cell membrane, resulting in a decreased sodium current. Among patients with these mutations there is a broad variability of symptom severity and age of onset leading to variable disease expression. There is also incomplete penetrance as some family members who have the same mutation may be asymptomatic. Conversely, patients with clinical Brugada Syndrome who have this mutation have family members who are not carriers of the same mutation but have a Brugada Syndrome typical ECG. It is unknown to this day whether the mutations in this cardiac sodium channel are causal or modify the severity of the disease. Due to the low diagnostic yield of genetic testing among clinically diagnosed Brugada syndrome patients (genetic abnormalities are found in about 30%), genetic testing is not recommended in the absence of a diagnostic ECG. Genetic testing may be useful for family members of a successfully genotyped proband. It should be noted that when considering genetic testing, a negative test cannot rule out Brugada Syndrome [38].

Prognosis and Risk Stratification

Brugada syndrome typically manifests during adulthood, with ventricular tachyarrhythmic events occurring at an average age of 40 years and sudden death typically occurring during rest or at sleep. Brugada syndrome is 8–10 times more prevalent in males than in females. At the time of diagnosis, males are more likely than females to present with previous symptoms, a spontaneous type I ECG pattern, and VF during an electrophysiology study (EPS) [39]. Although the basis for this sex-related distinction is unknown, it has been suggested that there is some sexual differences in gene expression or function and that the more prominent transient outward current (Ito) in males may contribute to the male predominance of the syndrome [40].

Currently, risk stratification in Brugada syndrome relies mainly on clinical factors. The most important clinical risk factor associated with high risk of life threatening arrhythmias is the presence of syncopal episodes in patients with a spontaneous type I ECG. Other risk factors include the presence of fragmented QRS, spontaneous atrial fibrillation, and ventricular effective refractory period <200 ms during an electrophysiology study (EPS) [41].

There is controversy regarding the value of programmed electrical stimulation during an EPS in predicting the risk for cardiac events. Brugada et al. [42] have found that inducibility of ventricular arrhythmias is a marker of a poor prognosis by multivariate analysis, but in both the PRELUDE (Programmed electrical stimulation predictive value) [7] and the FINGER (France, Italy, Netherlands, Germany) [43] registries, inducibility of sustained ventricular arrhythmias did not predict ventricular arrhythmic events by multivariate analysis. Family history of SCD was not found to be an independent risk factor for cardiac events.

There are limited data on how knowledge of the Brugada syndrome specific mutation may assist in risk stratification. The presence of an SCN5A mutation has not been proven to be a risk marker in Brugada syndrome, but non-missense mutations that result in a truncated protein or missense mutations with greater than 90% INa reduction have been found to predict syncopal episodes [44].

Management

The treatment of Brugada syndrome consists of lifestyle changes, ICD implantation and possibly medical therapy with Quinidine.

The expert consensus statement [3] recommends 3 lifestyle modifications for all patients with a diagnosis of Brugada syndrome: (1) avoidance of drugs that may induce or aggravate ST-segment elevation in the right precordial leads (avoiding some Ia and Ic antiarrhythmic drugs, several psychotropic drugs, and several anesthetics/analgesics including Propofol); (2) avoidance of excessive alcohol intake; and (3) immediate treatment of fever with antipyretic drugs.

ICD implantation is recommended for patients with a history of aborted cardiac arrest or spontaneous sustained VT for secondary prevention of SCD (class I indication). ICD can be useful for patients with a spontaneous type I ECG who have a history of syncope believed to result from VT. (Class IIa indication).

ICD implantation may be considered (Class IIb indication) in patients with Brugada syndrome and inducible VF during EPS.

Quinidine can be useful in patients who qualify for an ICD but have a contraindication for ICD implantation or refuse implantation. (Class IIa).

Quinidine may be considered (Class IIb) in asymptomatic patients with Brugada syndrome who have spontaneous type I ECG.

Patients with Brugada syndrome who experience arrhythmic storms (2 or more VT/VF episodes in 24 h) may be treated by quinidine, Isoproterenol (class IIa) or by catheter ablation targeting fractionated right ventricular electrograms (class IIb).

Technical Aspects

Procainamide Provocative Testing This provocative test may aid in unmasking individuals with Brugada syndrome. Baseline ECG (including high precordial leads) and vital signs should be taken at baseline, than start IV Procainamide 1 g over 30 min, measure vital signs and perform ECG every 10 min, stop infusion at 30 min and repeat ECG and vital signs at 40, 60, and 90 min. When performing provocative testing with a sodium channel blocker, the infusion should be terminated when a type- 1 ECG develops, premature ventricular beats or other arrhythmias develop, or the QRS widens to ≥130% of baseline [44].

Arrhythmogenic Right Ventricular Cardiomyopathy/Dysplasia (ARVC/D)

Incidence and Etiology

ARVC/D is a genetic heart muscle disease; its true prevalence is unknown, with estimates between 1 in 2000 and 1 in 5000. **This disorder is characterized by progressive myocyte loss with replacement by fatty or fibrous tissue and is associated with progressive ventricular dysfunction that may involve both ventricles** [45]. The resulting disruption of the RV myocardial architecture in ARVC/D can lead to RV dysfunction, ventricular tachyarrhythmias, syncope, or SCD [46]. The latter cardiac events may occur at a relative young age, particularly in the second and third decades of life, and often occurring during physical activity.

Syncope is reported in 16–39% of patients at the time of diagnosis and is frequently exercise related.

Several studies have suggested that mutations in various components of the cardiac desmosome have important roles in the pathogenesis of ARVC/D. Desmosomes are protein complexes specialized for cell-to-cell adhesion, supporting structural stability and maintaining normal electrical conductivity through regulation of gap junctions and calcium homeostasis. Defects in components of desmosomes may predispose to myocyte detachment and death, inflammation, repair by fibrofatty tissue, and life threatening ventricular arrhythmias [47].

Eight genes have been identified that are associated with ARVC/D: plakoglobin (JUP), desmoplakin (DSP), plakophilin-2 (PKP2), desmoglein-2 (DSG2), desmocollin-2 (DSC2), transforming growth factor beta-3 (TGFß3), ryanodine receptor 2 (RYR2) and TMEM. Five of these genes (plakoglobin, desmoplakin, desmoglein-2, plakophilin-2, and, desmocollin-2) encode major components of the cardiac desmosome. Currently known mutations in these genes identify 50% of patients with ARVC/D with the most common type of mutations reported are in the plakophilin-2 encoded gene.

Diagnosis

The diagnosis of ARVC/D is based on structural, histological, ECG, arrhythmic, and familial features of the disease. Abnormalities are subdivided into major and minor categories according to the specificity of their association with ARVC/D. The diagnosis of a definite ARVC/D is fulfilled by the presence of 2 major, or 1 major plus 2 minor criteria, or 4 minor criteria from different groups. According to a proposed modification of the International Task Force Criteria [8] there are 6 groups of criteria: (1) Global or regional dysfunction and structural alterations assessed by echocardiography, MRI or RV angiography; (2) Tissue characterization of wall assessed by endomyocardial biopsy and histopathology; (3) Repolarization abnormalities on the ECG including inverted T waves in right precordial leads; (4)

Depolarization/conduction abnormalities including Epsilon wave (low-amplitude signals between end of QRS complex to onset of the T wave in the right precordial leads) and late potentials by signal-averaged ECG; (5) Ventricular arrhythmias including nonsustained or sustained VT of left bundle-branch block morphology and .presence of >500 ventricular extrasystoles per 24 hours Holter monitoring; (6) Identification of a pathological mutation associated with ARVC/D or family history including a history of ARVC/D in a first-degree relative, or SCD at age < 35 years.

The yield of genetic testing in probands with suspected ARVC/D is about 30–54% and up to 58% among patients with a strong family history of SCD in multiple members, However, a negative genetic test does not exclude the disease [45].

As SCD can be the initial manifestation of ARVC/D, selected first-degree relatives could benefit from further screening and testing. Clinical screening with ECG, cardiac imaging and ambulatory rhythm monitoring and exercise testing may identify family members at risk for ARVC/D. This disorder is detected clinically in approximately 35–40% of first-degree relatives, more commonly in siblings or symptomatic first-degree relative. If a proband is identified with a disease causing mutation, genotype screening can identify genotype positive relatives. This is important as up to 35% of mutation positive individuals ultimately develop progressive disease expression.

Genotype-Phenotype Correlations and Risk Stratification

ARVC/D is inherited primarily in an autosomal dominant fashion, although there are recessive forms (e.g., Naxos disease, Carvajal syndrome) that are associated with a cutaneous phenotype. ARVC/D is a progressive heart muscle disease that with time may lead to more diffuse right ventricular (RV) involvement and left ventricular abnormalities. The severity of heart failure symptoms and the risk for ventricular arrhythmias vary considerably between patients.

There is controversy whether mutations in PKP2 (the most common implicated gene) are associated with poor prognosis and greater risk for arrhythmias [45, 48].

It was suggested that carriers of multiple mutations in ARVC/D-associated genes show a greater magnitude of myocardial involvement than carriers of a single mutation [49, 50].

In a large multicenter study, the presence of positive mutations among probands was not associated with a difference in mortality or cardiac transplantation. Identification of the pathogenic mutation, to date, provides limited prognostic information relative to the risk of VT/VF.

Genetic testing has an important role in the diagnosis of ARVC/D among symptomatic patients (a diagnostic yield of about 50%) and among relatives of genotype-positive patients.

Patients at increased risk for life threatening arrhythmic events include ARVC/D with extensive disease, including left ventricular involvement, history of syncope, and affected family members with SCD. In one study, syncope was an important predictor of appropriate shocks among patients with ARVC/D and implanted ICDs.

Sustained ventricular tachycardia is an important predictor of sudden cardiac arrest (SCA) and SCD or appropriate shocks in patients with ARVC/D. Additionally, frequent PVCs, >760 to 1000 per 24 h during ambulatory rhythm monitoring is associated with arrhythmic risk. The presence of NSVT or sustained VT is an important predictor of adverse cardiac events.

It is important to note that abnormal findings on signal averaged ECG correlate with disease severity on MRI and increased events in males. In fact, signal averaged ECG may be of greater value in the diagnosis of ARVC/D.

Management

Strenuous exercise should to be avoided. The increased risk with intense exercise is consistent with beta-adrenergic modulation of disease expression. In fact, vigorous exercise in these patients has been shown to impair myocardial function by echocardiography and MRI. Participation in high intensity or duration of physical activity accelerates the progression of the disease and its penetrance in mutation positive individuals. It is recommended to limit exercise intensity and duration to <650 MET-Hr/year or 12.5 MET-Hr/week.

Medical therapy used in this disorder consists of beta blockers and antiarrhythmic medications. An observational registry reported that treatment with atenolol or amiodarone was associated with less clinically relevant ventricular arrhythmias, while sotalol was associated with no effect or increased risk. However, in an observational series, sotalol suppressed inducible VT in 58% of patients with less than 10% of patients experiencing arrhythmia recurrence during follow up. More studies are necessary to elucidate the efficacy of medical treatment in ARVC/D. To date, there are no data that drug treatment improves survival in the absence of sustained ventricular arrhythmias [47].

Thus, the mainstay of treatment is ICD implantation in selected ARVC/D patients. There is consensus that patients who had sustained VT or aborted cardiac arrest should have an ICD (Class Ia indication) [9]. As sustained VT in this disorder is monomorphic in 55% to 90% of episodes based on ICD interrogation or electrophysiological studies, antitachycardia pacing algorithms are used to terminate VT.

The ACC/AHA/ESC guidelines also state that ARVC/D with extensive disease, including left ventricular involvement, one or more affected family members with SCD, or syncope are at greater risk and should receive an ICD [18].

Ablation is moderately successful for VT, but combined ICD treatment is necessary regardless of outcome. VT is usually related to scar-related reentry, and the sub epicardium usually has more extensive scar than the endocardium. In experienced centers, use of epicardial mapping and ablation is associated with better outcomes. Ablation reduces the frequency of recurrent VT, but 27% to 55% of patients have at least one recurrence. Occasional patients will undergo cardiac transplantation either because of intractable arrhythmias or severe heart failure.

Catecholaminergic Polymorphic Ventricular Tachycardia [51]

Catecholaminergic polymorphic ventricular tachycardia (CPVT) is a rare congenital arrhythmogenic disorder induced by physical exercise or emotional stress. The arrhythmias that characterize this disorder include polymorphic VT and bidirectional VT. It mainly affects younger children as the age of onset is usually 8 years old, but it can also affect infants and adults. The proportion of males vs females having this disorder is about the same, but there is a higher risk of CEs in males.

Genetics and Pathophysiology

The majority of CPVT cases are familial. However, the disorder can present spontaneously as a de novo mutation in patients without a family history of CPVT. There are several mutations that exist for CPVT but the two most common are in the genes for the cardiac ryanodine receptor (RyR2) and the calsequeststrin 2 (CASQ2).

The RyR2 mutation has autosomal dominant inheritance pattern and accounts for about 60–70% of CPVT cases. The CASQ2 mutation has autosomal recessive pattern and accounts for 10–15% of the cases. This gene mutation is typically more severe than the RyR2 mutation.

The propensity towards life-threatening ventricular tachyarrhythmias is associated with the inherited dysfunction in the calcium ion handling by the sarcoplasmic reticulum in cardiac myocytes. Under catecholaminergic stimulation, either mutation can result in an excess calcium load during diastole with a subsequent delayed after depolarization leading to arrhythmogenesis.

Clinical Presentation

The initial presentation may involve mild symptoms such as dizziness, paleness, lightheadedness and palpitations. As the burden and duration of this disorder worsens, patients may develop subsequent syncope, hypotonia, and even convulsions. Syncopal episodes can be very brief, and a failure to recognize them may lead to progression to SCD.

Symptoms are usually present only if there is a trigger such as physical activity or emotional stress. At rest, these patients would typically not have any abnormalities on diagnostic modalities.

Diagnosis

In order to diagnose CPVT, patients need to demonstrate polymorphic ventricular tachycardia induced by adrenergic stimulation in the absence of a structural heart disease and a normal EKG. The diagnostic tests that are usually carried out include either a 48 h Holter monitor or an exercise stress test. If the patient cannot exercise, a small infusion of isoproterenol to simulate physical stress. It is important to note that this disorder has incomplete penetrance and the first presentation of CPVT in a family member can be SCD. Therefore, screening even asymptomatic family members is very important.

Treatment

According to the 2013 Heart Rhythm Society, the European Heart Rhythm Association, and the Asia Pacific Heart Rhythm Society Expert Consensus Recommendations on CPVT Therapeutic Interventions, class I treatment recommendation involves: (1) Lifestyle modifications, (2) Beta blockers for symptomatic patients, (3) ICD implantation for CPVT patients experiencing life threatening episodes such as cardiac arrest, recurrent syncope, or polymorphic ventricular tachycardia despite medical management.

Lifestyle interventions typically involves limiting competitive sports and strenuous exercise. However, studies have shown that if patients remain asymptomatic on an optimal medical regimen, they can exercise with a relatively low risk for CEs. Risk factors for CEs in CPVT generally include the age of onset and noncompliance with a treatment regimen. Exercise may actually be important as it reduces the chances of obesity, diabetes, depression. Moderate exercise, in asymptomatic patients under a comprehensive treatment, may also improve cardiac function and may even attenuate exercise induced arrhythmias.

Life-long administration of beta-blockers is currently recommended as a first line treatment option for CPVT. The most commonly used drug is nadolol, both effective in treating symptoms and as a prophylactic agents. Beta blockers generally decrease the severity of arrhythmias experienced by these patients. However, while beta-blockers may prevent the onset of arrhythmias, a review of 11 past studies revealed that after 8 years, 6.4% of CPVT patients had a fatal event. This suggests that even though there is a reduction in cardiac arrhythmic events with beta-blockers, there is still a residual cardiac event rate even on patients who receive this treatment.

The main causes of failure of beta-blocker therapy include poor drug compliance or insufficient dosing. Generally, the highest tolerated dose of the beta blocker should be used, and in children, the dose should be titrated as the child grows. Beta blockers are key in the treatment of CPVT and due to their significant prophylactic effects, they should also be prescribed to genetically positive but asymptomatic family members of CPVT patients.

ICD is strongly recommended in patients with residual cardiac events despite appropriate beta blocker therapy. However, in CPVT the therapeutic benefits of the ICD are limited. In a comprehensive review of CPVT patients, only half the patients received an appropriate shock that was able to terminate the ventricular arrhythmia. Inappropriate shocks were very common and up to 22% of patients with CPVT received at least 1 inappropriate shocks. In this patient population, even an appropriate shock can have fatal outcomes, as an ICD shock can trigger catecholamine release and induce more ICD shocks resulting in a VT storm which may ultimately lead to death. For these reasons ICD implantation should be considered carefully in patients with CPVT. If a decision is made to implant the ICD, then higher detection zones should be used as well as longer detection times.

More recently, flecainide, was introduced as an adjunctive treatment in patients who have had CEs despite beta blocker use.

This class 1C antiarrhythmic works by blocking the RyR2 channel and suppressing calcium release from the SR, thereby targeting the mechanisms that lead to arrhythmias in CPVT. In one study, 85% of patients on a combined therapy had complete suppression of ventricular arrhythmias.

Left cardiac sympathetic denervation is recommended for patients who remain symptomatic despite the highest tolerable dose of beta blocker therapy. There are many studies that suggest that this method of arrhythmia suppression is highly effective, with up to 75% of CPVT patients who have undergone LCSD did not experience any cardiac events post denervation. This method, however, must be weighed against the postoperative side effects which can be common.

Other therapies that are not yet listed in guidelines and require further investigations include: calcium channel blockers, RyR2 channel blockers, and gene therapy.

Fabry Disease

Fabry disease (FD) is an X-linked lysosomal storage disorder caused by deficiency of alpha galactosidase A enzyme [52]. This leads to failure in the degradation of glycophospholipids and subsequently their lysosomal accumulation. This over time results in multi-system disease including progressive renal impairment, cardiomyopathy, and cerebrovascular events. There is significant variability in the presentation of this disease with "classical" males generally developing the severe form of the disease. Other phenotypes may be present in women, for example, who can present typically at a later age if heterozygous. There are also variants with predominant cardiac involvement known as the "cardiac variants".

Cardiovascular features of this disease may include left ventricular hypertrophy, congestive heart failure, and arrhythmia. Palpitations and syncope are common and have been reported in up to 30% of patients. In fact, cardiovascular disease is the most common cause of death in FD. Although it is difficult to determine causality, lysosomal accumulation of glycosphingolipids may affect conduction tissue and cardiomyocytes. These can lead to release of pro-inflammatory cytokines as well as pro-thrombotic factors and growth promotic factors which lead to oxidative stress and impaired cardiac metabolism. Ultimately the inflammation and tissue injury leads to ventricular arrhythmias via differing mechanisms including, vascular damage, cardiac remodeling, and direct damage to the cardiomyocytes.

A systematic review of FD found that up to 62% of reported deaths are due to SCD. A study of 1448 untreated Fabry patients showed ventricular arrhythmias in 13% of men and 20% of women.

Risk factors identified for SCD and VA include male gender, older age, increasing LV mass index, the presence of late gandolinium enhancement on MRI, and prior non-sustained ventricular tachycardia. The characteristic features of FD on cardiac MRI include the presence of LGE in the basal inferolateral left ventricle, which correlates with marked fibrosis on histology in this region in advanced disease. Unlike ischemic cardiomyopathy, it is possible the VA in FD develops from intramural or epicardial sites similar to other non-ischemic cardiomyopathies.

In a study it was found that 4.2% of FD patients needed an ICD due to non-sustained VT. Treatment of the cardiac manifestations of the disease should also focus on treatment of the underlying disease process. Recombinant alpha-galactosidase A has been approved since 2001. This mode of therapy should be initiated at the age of 16 years regardless of symptomatic status [53]. Another mode of therapy is migalastat which is a first in class pharmacological chaperone therapy for FD.

References

1. Schwartz PJ, Stramba-Badiale M, Crotti L, Pedrazzini M, Besana A, Bosi G, Gabbarini F, Goulene K, Insolia R, Mannarino S, Mosca F, Nespoli L, Rimini A, Rosati E, Salice P, Spazzolini C. Prevalence of the congenital long-QT syndrome. Circulation. 2009;120:1761–7.
2. Goldenberg I, Moss AJ. Long QT syndrome. J Am Coll Cardiol. 2008;51:2291–300.

3. Krahn AD, Laksman Z, Sy RW, Postema PG, Ackerman MJ, Wilde AAM, Han HC. Congenital long QT syndrome. JACC Clin Electrophysiol. 2022;8:687–706.
4. Neira V, Enriquez A, Simpson C, Baranchuk A. Update on long QT syndrome. J Cardiovasc Electrophysiol. 2019;30:3068–78.
5. Priori SG, Wilde AA, Horie M, Cho Y, Behr ER, Berul C, Blom N, Brugada J, Chiang CE, Huikuri H, Kannankeril P, Krahn A, Leenhardt A, Moss A, Schwartz PJ, Shimizu W, Tomaselli G, Tracy C. HRS/EHRA/APHRS expert consensus statement on the diagnosis and management of patients with inherited primary arrhythmia syndromes expert consensus statement on inherited primary arrhythmia syndromes: document endorsed by HRS, EHRA, and APHRS in May 2013 and by ACCF, AHA, PACES, and AEPC in June 2013. Heart Rhythm. 2013:e75–e106.
6. Schwartz PJ, Moss AJ, Vincent GM, Crampton RS. Diagnostic criteria for the long QT syndrome. An update. Circulation. 1993;88:782–4.
7. Goldenberg I, Horr S, Moss AJ, Lopes CM, Barsheshet A, McNitt S, Zareba W, Andrews ML, Robinson JL, Locati EH, Ackerman MJ, Benhorin J, Kaufman ES, Napolitano C, Platonov PG, Priori SG, Qi M, Schwartz PJ, Shimizu W, Towbin JA, Vincent GM, Wilde AA, Zhang L. Risk for life-threatening cardiac events in patients with genotype-confirmed long-QT syndrome and normal-range corrected QT intervals. J Am Coll Cardiol. 2011;57:51–9.
8. Viskin S, Postema PG, Bhuiyan ZA, Rosso R, Kalman JM, Vohra JK, Guevara-Valdivia ME, Marquez MF, Kogan E, Belhassen B, Glikson M, Strasberg B, Antzelevitch C, Wilde AA. The response of the QT interval to the brief tachycardia provoked by standing: a bedside test for diagnosing long QT syndrome. J Am Coll Cardiol. 2010;55:1955–61.
9. Horner JM, Horner MM, Ackerman MJ. The diagnostic utility of recovery phase QTc during treadmill exercise stress testing in the evaluation of long QT syndrome. Heart Rhythm. 2011;8:1698–704.
10. Vyas H, Hejlik J, Ackerman MJ. Epinephrine QT stress testing in the evaluation of congenital long-QT syndrome: diagnostic accuracy of the paradoxical QT response. Circulation. 2006;113:1385–92.
11. Viskin S, Rosso R, Rogowski O, Belhassen B, Levitas A, Wagshal A, Katz A, Fourey D, Zeltser D, Oliva A, Pollevick GD, Antzelevitch C, Rozovski U. Provocation of sudden heart rate oscillation with adenosine exposes abnormal QT responses in patients with long QT syndrome: a bedside test for diagnosing long QT syndrome. Eur Heart J. 2006;27:469–75.
12. Moss AJ, Zareba W, Benhorin J, Locati EH, Hall WJ, Robinson JL, Schwartz PJ, Towbin JA, Vincent GM, Lehmann MH. ECG T-wave patterns in genetically distinct forms of the hereditary long QT syndrome. Circulation. 1995;92:2929–34.

13. Ackerman MJ, Tester DJ, Porter CJ. Swimming, a gene-specific arrhythmogenic trigger for inherited long QT syndrome. Mayo Clin Proc. 1999;74:1088–94.
14. Moss AJ, Robinson JL, Gessman L, Gillespie R, Zareba W, Schwartz PJ, Vincent GM, Benhorin J, Heilbron EL, Towbin JA, Priori SG, Napolitano C, Zhang L, Medina A, Andrews ML, Timothy K. Comparison of clinical and genetic variables of cardiac events associated with loud noise versus swimming among subjects with the long QT syndrome. Am J Cardiol. 1999;84:876–9.
15. Costa J, Lopes CM, Barsheshet A, Moss AJ, Migdalovich D, Ouellet G, McNitt S, Polonsky S, Robinson JL, Zareba W, Ackerman MJ, Benhorin J, Kaufman ES, Platonov PG, Shimizu W, Towbin JA, Vincent GM, Wilde AA, Goldenberg I. Combined assessment of sex- and mutation-specific information for risk stratification in type 1 long QT syndrome. Heart Rhythm. 2012;9:892–8.
16. Migdalovich D, Moss AJ, Lopes CM, Costa J, Ouellet G, Barsheshet A, McNitt S, Polonsky S, Robinson JL, Zareba W, Ackerman MJ, Benhorin J, Kaufman ES, Platonov PG, Shimizu W, Towbin JA, Vincent GM, Wilde AA, Goldenberg I. Mutation and gender-specific risk in type 2 long QT syndrome: implications for risk stratification for life-threatening cardiac events in patients with long QT syndrome. Heart Rhythm. 2011;8:1537–43.
17. Goldenberg I, Bos JM, Yoruk A, Chen AY, Lopes C, Huang DT, Kutyifa V, Younis A, Aktas MK, Rosero SZ, McNitt S, Sotoodehnia N, Kudenchuk PJ, Rea TD, Arking DE, Scott CG, Briske KA, Sorensen K, Ackerman MJ, Zareba W. Risk prediction in women with congenital long QT syndrome. J Am Heart Assoc. 2021;10:e021088.
18. Goldenberg I, Younis A, Huang DT, Yoruk A, Rosero SZ, Cutter K, Kutyifa V, McNitt S, Sotoodehnia N, Kudenchuk PJ, Rea TD, Arking DE, Polonski B, Zareba W, Aktas MK. Use of oral contraceptives in women with congenital long QT syndrome. Heart Rhythm. 2022;19:41–8.
19. Mullally J, Goldenberg I, Moss AJ, Lopes CM, Ackerman MJ, Zareba W, McNitt S, Robinson JL, Benhorin J, Kaufman ES, Towbin JA, Barsheshet A. Risk of life-threatening cardiac events among patients with long QT syndrome and multiple mutations. Heart Rhythm. 2013;10:378–82.
20. Zipes DP, Camm AJ, Borggrefe M, Buxton AE, Chaitman B, Fromer M, Gregoratos G, Klein G, Moss AJ, Myerburg RJ, Priori SG, Quinones MA, Roden DM, Silka MJ, Tracy C, Smith SC Jr, Jacobs AK, Adams CD, Antman EM, Anderson JL, Hunt SA, Halperin JL, Nishimura R, Ornato JP, Page RL, Riegel B, Priori SG, Blanc JJ, Budaj A, Camm AJ, Dean V, Deckers JW, Despres C, Dickstein K, Lekakis J, McGregor K, Metra M, Morais J, Osterspey A, Tamargo JL, Zamorano JL. ACC/AHA/ESC 2006 guidelines for management of patients with ventricular arrhythmias and the prevention of sudden cardiac death: a report of the American College of Cardiology/American Heart Association Task Force and the European

Society of Cardiology Committee for Practice Guidelines (writing committee to develop guidelines for management of patients with ventricular arrhythmias and the prevention of sudden cardiac death). J Am Coll Cardiol. 2006;48:e247-346.
21. Kim JA, Lopes CM, Moss AJ, McNitt S, Barsheshet A, Robinson JL, Zareba W, Ackerman MJ, Kaufman ES, Towbin JA, Vincent M, Goldenberg I. Trigger-specific risk factors and response to therapy in long QT syndrome type 2. Heart Rhythm. 2010;7:1797–805.
22. Schwartz PJ, Priori SG, Spazzolini C, Moss AJ, Vincent GM, Napolitano C, Denjoy I, Guicheney P, Breithardt G, Keating MT, Towbin JA, Beggs AH, Brink P, Wilde AA, Toivonen L, Zareba W, Robinson JL, Timothy KW, Corfield V, Wattanasirichaigoon D, Corbett C, Haverkamp W, Schulze-Bahr E, Lehmann MH, Schwartz K, Coumel P, Bloise R. Genotype-phenotype correlation in the long-QT syndrome: gene-specific triggers for life-threatening arrhythmias. Circulation. 2001;103:89–95.
23. Moss AJ, Zareba W, Hall WJ, Schwartz PJ, Crampton RS, Benhorin J, Vincent GM, Locati EH, Priori SG, Napolitano C, Medina A, Zhang L, Robinson JL, Timothy K, Towbin JA, Andrews ML. Effectiveness and limitations of beta-blocker therapy in congenital long-QT syndrome. Circulation. 2000;101:616–23.
24. Goldenberg I, Bradley J, Moss A, McNitt S, Polonsky S, Robinson JL, Andrews M, Zareba W. Beta-blocker efficacy in high-risk patients with the congenital long-QT syndrome types 1 and 2: implications for patient management. J Cardiovasc Electrophysiol. 2010;21:893–901.
25. Barsheshet A, Goldenberg I, O-Uchi J, Moss AJ, Jons C, Shimizu W, Wilde AA, McNitt S, Peterson DR, Zareba W, Robinson JL, Ackerman MJ, Cypress M, Gray DA, Hofman N, Kanters JK, Kaufman ES, Platonov PG, Qi M, Towbin JA, Vincent GM, Lopes CM. Mutations in cytoplasmic loops of the KCNQ1 channel and the risk of life-threatening events: implications for mutation-specific response to beta-blocker therapy in type 1 long-QT syndrome. Circulation. 2012;125:1988–96.
26. Matavel A, Medei E, Lopes CM. PKA and PKC partially rescue long QT type 1 phenotype by restoring channel-PIP(2) interactions. Channels (Austin). 2010;4.
27. Chockalingam P, Crotti L, Girardengo G, Johnson JN, Harris KM, van der Heijden JF, Hauer RN, Beckmann BM, Spazzolini C, Rordorf R, Rydberg A, Clur SA, Fischer M, van den Heuvel F, Kaab S, Blom NA, Ackerman MJ, Schwartz PJ, Wilde AA. Not all beta-blockers are equal in the management of long QT syndrome types 1 and 2: higher recurrence of events under metoprolol. J Am Coll Cardiol. 2012;60:2092.
28. Compton SJ, Lux RL, Ramsey MR, Strelich KR, Sanguinetti MC, Green LS, Keating MT, Mason JW. Genetically defined therapy of inherited long-QT syndrome. Correction of abnormal repolarization by potassium. Circulation. 1996;94:1018–22.

29. Etheridge SP, Compton SJ, Tristani-Firouzi M, Mason JW. A new oral therapy for long QT syndrome: long-term oral potassium improves repolarization in patients with HERG mutations. J Am Coll Cardiol. 2003;42:1777–82.
30. Schwartz PJ, Priori SG, Locati EH, Napolitano C, Cantu F, Towbin JA, Keating MT, Hammoude H, Brown AM, Chen LS. Long QT syndrome patients with mutations of the SCN5A and HERG genes have differential responses to Na+ channel blockade and to increases in heart rate. Implications for gene-specific therapy. Circulation. 1995;92:3381–6.
31. Nagatomo T, January CT, Makielski JC. Preferential block of late sodium current in the LQT3 DeltaKPQ mutant by the class I(C) antiarrhythmic flecainide. Mol Pharmacol. 2000;57:101–7.
32. Windle JR, Geletka RC, Moss AJ, Zareba W, Atkins DL. Normalization of ventricular repolarization with flecainide in long QT syndrome patients with SCN5A:DeltaKPQ mutation. Ann Noninvasive Electrocardiol. 2001;6:153–8.
33. Roston TM, van der Werf C, Cheung CC, Grewal J, Davies B, Wilde AAM, Krahn AD. Caring for the pregnant woman with an inherited arrhythmia syndrome. Heart Rhythm. 2020;17:341–8.
34. Moss AJ, Windle JR, Hall WJ, Zareba W, Robinson JL, McNitt S, Severski P, Rosero S, Daubert JP, Qi M, Cieciorka M, Manalan AS. Safety and efficacy of flecainide in subjects with long QT-3 syndrome (DeltaKPQ mutation): a randomized, double-blind, placebo-controlled clinical trial. Ann Noninvasive Electrocardiol. 2005;10:59–66.
35. Stokoe KS, Balasubramaniam R, Goddard CA, Colledge WH, Grace AA, Huang CL. Effects of flecainide and quinidine on arrhythmogenic properties of Scn5a+/− murine hearts modelling the Brugada syndrome. J Physiol. 2007;581:255–75.
36. Anno T, Hondeghem LM. Interactions of flecainide with Guinea pig cardiac sodium channels. Importance of activation unblocking to the voltage dependence of recovery. Circ Res. 1990;66:789–803.
37. Goldenberg I, Moss AJ, Zareba W. QT interval: how to measure it and what is "normal". J Cardiovasc Electrophysiol. 2006;17:333–6.
38. Marsman EMJ, Postema PG, Remme CA. Brugada syndrome: update and future perspectives. Heart. 2022;108:668–75.
39. Brugada P, Brugada J. Right bundle branch block, persistent ST segment elevation and sudden cardiac death: a distinct clinical and electrocardiographic syndrome. A multicenter report. J Am Coll Cardiol. 1992;20:1391–6.
40. Benito B, Sarkozy A, Mont L, Henkens S, Berruezo A, Tamborero D, Arzamendi D, Berne P, Brugada R, Brugada P, Brugada J. Gender differences in clinical manifestations of Brugada syndrome. J Am Coll Cardiol. 2008;52:1567–73.
41. Marcus FI, McKenna WJ, Sherrill D, Basso C, Bauce B, Bluemke DA, Calkins H, Corrado D, Cox MG, Daubert JP, Fontaine G, Gear K, Hauer

R, Nava A, Picard MH, Protonotarios N, Saffitz JE, Sanborn DM, Steinberg JS, Tandri H, Thiene G, Towbin JA, Tsatsopoulou A, Wichter T, Zareba W. Diagnosis of arrhythmogenic right ventricular cardiomyopathy/ dysplasia: proposed modification of the task force criteria. Circulation. 2010;121:1533–41.
42. Awad MM, Calkins H, Judge DP. Mechanisms of disease: molecular genetics of arrhythmogenic right ventricular dysplasia/cardiomyopathy. Nat Clin Pract Cardiovasc Med. 2008;5:258–67.
43. Priori SG, Gasparini M, Napolitano C, Della Bella P, Ottonelli AG, Sassone B, Giordano U, Pappone C, Mascioli G, Rossetti G, De Nardis R, Colombo M. Risk stratification in Brugada syndrome: results of the PRELUDE (PRogrammed ELectrical stimUlation preDictive valuE) registry. J Am Coll Cardiol. 2012;59:37–45.
44. Meregalli PG, Tan HL, Probst V, Koopmann TT, Tanck MW, Bhuiyan ZA, Sacher F, Kyndt F, Schott JJ, Albuisson J, Mabo P, Bezzina CR, Le Marec H, Wilde AA. Type of SCN5A mutation determines clinical severity and degree of conduction slowing in loss-of-function sodium channelopathies. Heart Rhythm. 2009;6:341–8.
45. Al-Khatib SM, Stevenson WG, Ackerman MJ, Bryant WJ, Callans DJ, Curtis AB, Deal BJ, Dickfeld T, Field ME, Fonarow GC, Gillis AM, Granger CB, Hammill SC, Hlatky MA, Joglar JA, Kay GN, Matlock DD, Myerburg RJ, Page RL. 2017 AHA/ACC/HRS guideline for management of patients with ventricular arrhythmias and the prevention of sudden cardiac death. Circulation. 2018;138:e272–391.
46. Marcus FI, Zareba W, Calkins H, Towbin JA, Basso C, Bluemke DA, Estes NA 3rd, Picard MH, Sanborn D, Thiene G, Wichter T, Cannom D, Wilber DJ, Scheinman M, Duff H, Daubert J, Talajic M, Krahn A, Sweeney M, Garan H, Sakaguchi S, Lerman BB, Kerr C, Kron J, Steinberg JS, Sherrill D, Gear K, Brown M, Severski P, Polonsky S, McNitt S. Arrhythmogenic right ventricular cardiomyopathy/dysplasia clinical presentation and diagnostic evaluation: results from the north American Multidisciplinary Study. Heart Rhythm. 2009;6:984–92.
47. Dalal D, Molin LH, Piccini J, Tichnell C, James C, Bomma C, Prakasa K, Towbin JA, Marcus FI, Spevak PJ, Bluemke DA, Abraham T, Russell SD, Calkins H, Judge DP. Clinical features of arrhythmogenic right ventricular dysplasia/cardiomyopathy associated with mutations in plakophilin-2. Circulation. 2006;113:1641–9.
48. van Tintelen JP, Entius MM, Bhuiyan ZA, Jongbloed R, Wiesfeld AC, Wilde AA, van der Smagt J, Boven LG, Mannens MM, van Langen IM, Hofstra RM, Otterspoor LC, Doevendans PA, Rodriguez LM, van Gelder IC, Hauer RN. Plakophilin-2 mutations are the major determinant of familial arrhythmogenic right ventricular dysplasia/cardiomyopathy. Circulation. 2006;113:1650–8.
49. Bauce B, Nava A, Beffagna G, Basso C, Lorenzon A, Smaniotto G, De Bortoli M, Rigato I, Mazzotti E, Steriotis A, Marra MP, Towbin JA,

Thiene G, Danieli GA, Rampazzo A. Multiple mutations in desmosomal proteins encoding genes in arrhythmogenic right ventricular cardiomyopathy/dysplasia. Heart Rhythm. 2010;7:22–9.
50. Smith W. Guidelines for the diagnosis and management of arrhythmogenic right ventricular cardiomyopathy. Heart Lung Circ. 2011;20:757–60.
51. Kim CW, Aronow WS, Dutta T, Frenkel D, Frishman WH. Catecholaminergic polymorphic ventricular tachycardia. Cardiol Rev. 2020;28:325–31.
52. Baig S, Edward NC, Kotecha D, Liu B, Nordin S, Kozor R, Moon JC, Geberhiwot T, Steeds RP. Ventricular arrhythmia and sudden cardiac death in Fabry disease: a systematic review of risk factors in clinical practice. Europace. 2018;20:f153–61.
53. Mahmud HM. Fabry's disease—a comprehensive review on pathogenesis, diagnosis and treatment. J Pak Med Assoc. 2014;64:189–94.

Index

A

Ablation, 28, 38, 55, 65, 85–88, 91–97, 99, 110, 112–116, 118–127, 132, 134, 136–138, 141–146, 148–156, 159–169, 173, 180, 190–192, 194, 195, 197–199, 202, 203, 205–207, 209–210, 212–214, 216, 243

Accessory pathways, 92, 96, 105, 113, 115, 119

Activation mapping, 115, 138, 146, 165, 199, 205, 206

Arrhythmogenic right ventricular cardiomyopathy/dysplasia (ARVC/D), 239–243

Atrial fibrillation, 4, 16, 20, 24–28, 43, 44, 49, 54, 55, 65, 71, 78, 93, 104, 105, 108–114, 126, 130–132, 143, 148, 149, 152–156, 172, 237

Atrial flutter, 76, 90, 93, 97, 130–137, 139, 141, 142, 144, 152

Atrial tachycardia, 44, 82, 87–94, 97, 105, 131

Atrioventricular nodal reentrant tachycardia, 82–87, 93, 95–96, 104, 105

Atrioventricular (AV) node, 2, 3, 5–11, 48, 64, 83, 86, 88, 92, 105, 106, 112, 113, 123–125, 193

Atypical atrial flutter, 90, 132, 133, 143

B

Bradycardia, 4, 5, 20, 24, 25, 27, 33, 35, 38, 41, 48, 49, 137, 223, 233

Brugada, 182, 183, 209, 234–239

C

Cardiac anatomy, 173

Cardiac arrest, 53, 112, 226, 228, 232, 235, 236, 238, 242, 243, 245

Cardiac conduction, 5, 9, 12, 32, 48, 49

Cardiac devices therapy, 47–78

Cardiac resynchronization therapy (CRT), 54, 55

Cardioversion, 32–36, 38, 40–44, 114

Index

Catheter ablation, 55, 85, 112, 136, 154–156, 172, 173, 189, 191, 209, 210, 215, 239
Cryoballoon, 153, 168–172

D
Defibrillation threshold testing (DFT), 54
Dual loop flutter, 133–135, 139

E
ECG, *see* Electrocardiogram
Electroanatomic mapping, 2, 3, 96, 139, 145, 160, 167, 211
Electrocardiogram (ECG), 2–11, 16, 17, 20, 23, 25–28, 82, 84, 87, 89–92, 104, 105, 116, 118, 126, 141, 153, 182, 184, 186, 191, 194, 196, 199, 200, 203, 204, 207, 208, 211, 220, 222, 224, 232, 234–242
Entrainment mapping, 193–195, 198
Epicardial access, 191, 200
Event monitor, 16, 19–23, 28, 85

F
Fabry disease, 247

H
Heart block, 4–6, 8, 11, 12, 49
Hereditary arrhythmias, 220
His bundle, 2, 5, 6, 9, 10, 48, 65, 66, 87, 88, 95, 193, 206, 209
His bundle pacing, 65–67
Holter monitor, 16–20, 28, 49, 149, 153, 211, 241, 245

I
Impendence, 52, 71
Implantable cardiac defibrillator, 59–61
Implantable loop recorders (ILR), 16, 25, 35, 38, 49, 153
Interrogation, 53, 68–70, 243
Intracardiac echo, 124, 154, 156, 193

L
Left bundle branch pacing, 67–68
Long QT Syndrome (LQTS), 220, 226, 232

M
Macroreentrant tachycardia, 97
Mobile continuous outpatient telemetry (MCOT), 16, 23, 24

O
Orthodromic tachycardia, 104, 105, 113, 115, 119, 123, 124
Orthostatic hypotension, 35–36, 39, 40

P
Pacemaker, 4–6, 9, 10, 16, 35, 38, 44, 49, 50, 54, 56, 60–64, 71, 73, 137, 233
Pacing maneuvers, 9, 87, 92, 97, 188
Palpitations, 18, 24, 85, 90, 104, 149, 244, 247
Postablation, 156
Preexcited atrial fibrillation, 105, 108, 109, 112, 114, 125–126

Index

Pulmonary vein isolation (PVI), 142, 148, 168, 169, 172–173

R
Radiofrequency, 91, 142, 151–153, 158, 160–168, 173, 202, 207
Reflex syncope, 34, 35

S
Sensing, 52, 54, 60–62, 69–73, 124, 214
Sinus node, 2–5, 7, 9, 43–44, 48, 49, 64, 89, 90
Smartwatches, 27
Substrate modification, 199
Sudden cardiac death (SCD), 16, 53, 180, 209, 226
Supraventricular tachycardia, 16, 82, 83, 85–88, 90, 91, 93–97, 99, 100
Syncope, 4, 5, 8, 18, 24, 32–38, 40, 41, 43, 44, 48, 49, 108, 187, 220, 224, 225, 228, 235, 238, 240, 242, 243, 245, 247

T
Tachycardia, 20, 24, 25, 27, 33, 44, 55, 82–85, 87, 88, 90, 91, 105, 121, 123, 138, 182, 186, 195, 208
3D mapping, 88, 91, 93–95, 97, 115, 198, 205, 210, 211
Threshold, 5, 52, 54, 58, 60, 66, 70, 71, 73, 151
Tilt table testing, 32–36, 38–41, 43, 44
Torsades de Pointes, 224
Typical atrial flutter, 132, 133, 138, 142

V
Ventricular fibrillation, 8, 43, 108, 109, 189, 193, 209–210
Ventricular preexcitation, 104
Ventricular tachyarrhthmia, 180, 182, 216, 232, 237, 239, 244
Ventricular tachycardia, 8, 44, 55, 71, 181, 182, 187–194, 203, 204, 209, 215–216, 220, 242, 245, 248

W
Wolff-Parkinson-White Syndrome, 82

Printed in the United States
by Baker & Taylor Publisher Services